Concise Haematology

Concise Haematology

H. J. Woodliff
E.D., M.D., Ph.D., F.R.C.P.(E.), F.R.C.P.(A.)
Professor of Haematology
Makerere University, Uganda

and

R. P. Herrmann
M.B., M.R.A.C.P.
Assistant Haematologist
Royal Perth Hospital
Perth, Western Australia

The Williams & Wilkins Company
Baltimore

Edward Arnold

First published 1973
by Edward Arnold (Publishers) Ltd.
25 Hill Street,
London W1X 8LL

Boards Edition ISBN: 0 7131 4209 X
Paper Edition ISBN: 0 7131 4210 3

Printed in Great Britain by
T. and A. Constable Ltd, Edinburgh

Preface

Haematology is the study of the blood and blood-forming tissues and, as such, forms a separate branch of medical science. However, different aspects of the subject also form branches of other medical sciences: physiologists and biochemists are interested in the normal production, composition and destruction of the blood; clinical pathologists in the methods and value of examination of the blood and blood-forming tissues in the diagnosis and treatment of the disease; physicians in the management of patients with haematological disorders; and surgeons in the value of blood, its products or substitutes in preventing and treating 'shock'.

In this elementary account an attempt is made to integrate these different outlooks and present the subject as a whole. It is intended as an introduction to the subject suitable for medical students and practitioners who wish to use a separate text on haematology. It is not sufficiently comprehensive for postgraduate students who may find it helpful to them as a primer.

Normal blood production, composition and destruction are described and methods used in haematology are also considered but without technical details. Normal and disordered erythropoiesis, leucopoiesis, thrombopoiesis and haemostasis are then considered and there is a final section on blood groups and blood transfusion.

An attempt has been made to describe how the various abnormalities come about as well as giving the clinical and laboratory features of the more common disorders.

Greater detail than is given here can usually be obtained from the larger haematology textbooks or by consulting the bibliography given at the end of each chapter.

There are two large textbooks for the haematology specialist; a British book edited by Britton and an American one by Wintrobe. Both are too long for the general reader but are valuable reference books. Of interest to a wider audience is the textbook of clinical haematology by Professor de Gruchy, which can be recommended to trainee physicians and haematologists. There are several books dealing with the technical aspects of haematology which are suitable for those performing tests. These and several recommended atlases are listed at the end of Chapter 1.

Monographs on special subjects are available and some of these are listed at the end of the appropriate chapters.

H. J. W. wishes to thank his colleagues, teachers and students in Edinburgh, London and Cambridge who influenced his studies in haematology when this book had its beginnings as a series of notes. These were developed further at Oxford during the tenure of a lectureship where the guidance of Dr. A. A. Sharp is gratefully acknowledged.

During the last decade the lecture notes have been available to students in Western Australia. The task of revision, elaboration and preparation for publication has been undertaken by R. P. H.

We wish to thank our colleagues in Perth, Western Australia, especially Mr. R. E. Davis, Dr. M. G. Davey and Dr. J. M. Jackson, and in Kampala, Uganda Dr. S. Amsel and Dr. E. Nzaro for their many suggestions and for reading the manuscript.

Dr. L. Lajtha kindly agreed to the use of Fig. 2.1. The figures were prepared by Mrs. M. Blanchard.

Our thanks also to Mrs. J. Ritchie and Mrs. M. I. Woodliff who provided valuable secretarial assistance.

H. J. WOODLIFF
R. P. HERRMANN

LONDON, January 1973

Contents

1 Introduction and methods of study

COMPOSITION OF THE BLOOD

The heart and blood vessels of an adult human being contains about 5 litres of blood. This is made up of cells suspended in a fluid called plasma. The colour of the blood is due to the erythrocytes, or red cells, which contain the pigment haemoglobin; also present are leucocytes, or white cells, and thrombocytes, or platelets.

Serum and plasma

When blood is removed from the body and allowed to stand in a glass container for a few minutes, it clots. This is due to the precipitation of a soluble plasma protein, called fibrinogen, into strands of insoluble fibrin. The cells are caught up in a network of fibrin which gradually contracts, expressing a clear fluid called serum. Serum differs from plasma in not containing fibrinogen and in the concentration of some of the other substances concerned in the clotting mechanism.

Blood can be prevented from clotting by mixing it with anticoagulants which neutralize or remove some clotting factors. Plasma can be separated by allowing the cells to sediment or by centrifugation. It is a complex solution of proteins, salts, and other substances in water, and it may be opalescent due to the presence of fatty substances. Unless the specimen has been heavily centrifuged, some cells may remain in the plasma. The chemical composition of the plasma is not usually studied in haematology, except for substances concerned in blood production, conservation or destruction. These include iron, vitamins such as cobalamins and folates, the proteins needed for blood coagulation, free haemoglobin, haemoglobin derivatives, haptoglobins and transferrin.

Cytology

The cells in the blood are of three types: the erythrocytes, the leucocytes and the thrombocytes (platelets).

The erythrocytes, or red cells, are small biconcave discs without nuclei. They contain the pigment, haemoglobin, which combines loosely with oxygen, allowing it to be transported round the body. They are the most frequent cells in the blood, forming about 45% of its volume.

The leucocytes, or white cells, do not contain pigment. They are usually larger than the erythrocytes and contain nuclei. Three series of cells—granulocytes, lymphocytes and monocytes—are recognized. All are concerned in the defence of the body against infection. They form less than 1% of the blood volume.

The thrombocytes, or platelets, are very small and do not contain nuclei. They are concerned with the prevention of blood loss, both by 'blocking' holes in capillary blood vessels and by liberating coagulation factors when in contact with damaged tissues. They also form less than 1% of the blood by volume.

The peripheral blood cells are described in more detail in Chapters 1 and 2.

Sites of haemopoiesis

In the early fetus the process of haemopoiesis, as blood formation is called, takes place in the yolk sac and then in the liver and spleen. Later on, the bone marrow gradually replaces the liver and spleen as the site of erythropoiesis, granulopoiesis and thrombopoiesis. Lymphocytes are formed in the lymph nodes, in the spleen and in lymphatic tissues elsewhere in the body. Monocytes are produced in the reticuloendothelial tissues throughout the body, but particularly in the bone marrow, spleen and lymph nodes. After birth, the bone marrow is the only tissue producing erythrocytes, granulocytes and thrombocytes, but in some disorders this function is regained by the liver, the spleen and, occasionally, by the lymph nodes. This process is called extramedullary haemopoiesis.

Haemopoietic marrow is red. It fills most of the bone cavities at birth, but gradually it occupies relatively less of the available space, being replaced by non-haemopoietic marrow which is yellow due to the presence of fat. In the adult, red marrow is usually found in the flat bones and in the ends of the long bones. If there is an increase in blood production the volume of red marrow is increased by expansion in the long bones.

Disorders of the blood

Abnormalities of the blood cells are found in many diseases and are particularly marked in disorders of the haemopoietic tissues. Since one of the cell series is often more obviously affected than the others the disorders which occur can be conveniently divided into those affecting the erythrocytes, the leucocytes and the thrombocytes. It must be remembered, however, that this division is only one of emphasis and that in many of the disorders more than one cell series is involved. The relationship between cells and the plasma may also be altered. Abnormalities of the plasma are also found in many diseases. Of special interest to haematologists are defects of the coagulation factors, and these are considered separately. Other methods of classifying the blood disorders may be used; for example, into deficiency states, reactive processes and neoplasia. Before considering these in detail, it is necessary to consider some of the methods used in haematology.

METHODS OF STUDY

A large number of techniques are used in the study of blood and blood-forming tissues. The more common tests discussed in this section are listed in Table 1.1. Other tests of value in the investigation of particular blood

Table 1.1. Commonly requested blood tests

Haemoglobin estimation
Blood film
Haematocrit
Red cell count (automated)
White cell count
Differential white cell count
Erythrocyte sedimentation rate
Reticulocyte count
Platelet count

disorders are listed in Table 1.2; they are considered later in the appropriate chapter. Details of the methods used can be obtained from the practical manuals listed at the end of the chapter.

Collection of blood

If only a small quantity of blood is required, it may be obtained by pricking the skin of the finger or lobe of the ear with a sharp instrument. In infants blood is obtained from the heel. The skin is first cleaned with alcohol and allowed to dry. A sterile needle or lancet is inserted sharply into the skin to a depth of 1 or 2 mm. The first drop of blood to exude from the wound is wiped away with cotton wool. Subsequent drops are collected either on to a slide for a film or into a pipette or other container for various tests.

Blood in quantities greater than 0·5 ml should be collected from a vein. Generally speaking, venous blood is preferable for most examinations because, as well as allowing a larger specimen to be collected, it is less likely to be contaminated with tissue juices and the results of analyses on such specimens are more consistent than on capillary blood. An arm vein is usually used. After applying light pressure to the upper arm to retard venous return, a suitable vein is selected and the skin over it is wiped with alcohol. After the alcohol has evaporated a sharp, sterile needle, to which

Table 1.2. Other haematological tests

Bone marrow biopsy, aspiration or trephine
Examination for LE cells
Spectroscopy of plasma for abnormal pigments
Plasma haemoglobin
Schumm's test
Osmotic fragility of red cells
Mechanical fragility of red cells
Autohaemolysis test
Glucose-6-phosphate dehydrogenase, screening tests and assay
Stain for Heinz bodies
Ham's acid serum lysis test
Donath–Landsteiner antibody test
Test for cold agglutinins
Direct antiglobulin (Coombs') test
Urinary haemoglobin and urinary haemosiderin
Serum iron and total iron-binding capacity
Serum vitamin B_{12}
Absorption studies using ^{57}Co-labelled vitamin B_{12}
Serum folic acid
Red cell mass and plasma volume
Red cell survival using ^{51}Cr-labelled red cells
Plasma ^{59}Fe disappearance and red cell ^{59}Fe uptake
Platelet survival using ^{51}Cr-labelled platelets
Haemoglobin electrophoresis
Alkali-denaturation of haemoglobin to determine HbF
Sickling tests for HbS
Haemoglobin heat precipitation test
Oxygen-dissociation curve of blood

is attached a suitable-sized sterile syringe, is pushed through the skin and into the vein. Slight negative pressure on the barrel allows blood to be drawn into the syringe. When a sufficient quantity has been obtained the pressure on the upper arm is released and the needle withdrawn. Sterile cotton wool is applied to the puncture site with firm pressure for half a minute or so to prevent leakage of blood into the tissues. The needle should be removed from the syringe before distributing the blood into the specimen tubes.

Anticoagulants

If serum is required, the blood can be transferred directly into a sterile specimen tube. If whole blood or plasma is needed, an anticoagulant must be used. The most commonly used anticoagulant for specimen collection used to be the oxalate mixture of Heller and Paul. This consists of 4 mg of potassium oxalate and 6 mg of ammonium oxalate for each 5 ml of blood. This mixture was designed to prevent changes of red cells due to osmosis and is suitable for most haematological examinations. In many laboratories, however, it has been replaced by dipotassium EDTA (ethylenediamine tetra-acetic acid) in a concentration of 1–2 mg/ml of blood. Sodium citrate 3·8 % w/v is also used as an anticoagulant in the collection of blood for coagulation studies and for the Westergren erythrocyte sedimentation rate (ESR) measurement. One volume of anticoagulant is used for each five to ten volumes of blood. These three anticoagulants all act by 'binding' available calcium ions which are necessary for coagulation.

Heparin, an antithrombin anticoagulant, is used for special purposes when the removal of calcium is undesirable.

Haemoglobin concentration

The haemoglobin concentration in the blood can be measured in several ways. Analysis of the iron content is probably the most accurate method. However, it is too laborious for routine use and is used only for producing standards. The oxygen-binding capacity of blood gives a functional measurement of haemoglobin concentration but it also is too time consuming for general use.

Generally haemoglobin concentration is measured by comparing the colour of diluted blood with a standard. In such colorimetric methods the blood is usually treated in some way so that a single haemoglobin compound or derivative is present. Simpler screening tests are also sometimes used in field studies or when other facilities are not available; one such test, the copper sulphate specific gravity method, is mentioned later (p. 8).

The iron content

The iron content is measured by titrating a specially treated sample with titaneous chloride. The haemoglobin content is calculated from the formula that 1 g of haemoglobin contains 3·47 mg of iron.

The oxygen-combining capacity

The oxygen-combining capacity of blood is obtained by measuring the oxygen content of a fully saturated sample. The haemoglobin is worked out from the fact that 1 g of haemoglobin can combine with 1·37 ml of oxygen. The results obtained by this method are slightly lower than those obtained by iron analysis because only active oxygen-combining pigment is included.

Colorimetric methods

In colorimetric methods advantage is taken of the fact that haemoglobin can be converted into a variety of coloured compounds which can then be compared with various standards. The methods vary in accuracy, depending upon the method of comparison and the nature of the compound used and its standards.

Methods of comparison

Photo-electric absorptionometers (Fig. 1.1) provide the best means of measuring the light-absorbing capacities of coloured solutions. They are in universal use in hospital laboratories for haemoglobin estimations. The amount of light absorbed by a known dilution of treated blood is recorded on a galvanometer and the reading converted into grammes of haemoglobin

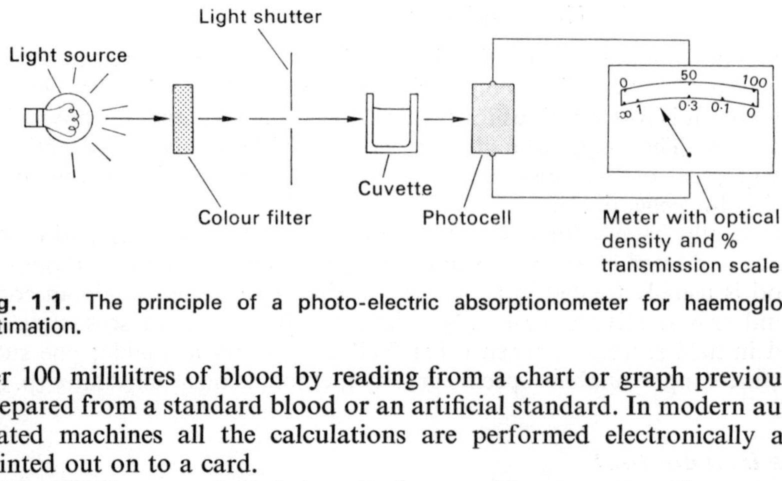

Fig. 1.1. The principle of a photo-electric absorptionometer for haemoglobin estimation.

per 100 millilitres of blood by reading from a chart or graph previously prepared from a standard blood or an artificial standard. In modern automated machines all the calculations are performed electronically and printed out on to a card.

The MRC grey-wedge photometer is a good instrument not incorporating a photo-electric cell (Fig. 1.2). The light absorbed by the haemoglobin solution is compared with that absorbed by a neutral grey wedge.

Older methods (for example, those of Haldane and Sahli) which depend upon the progressive dilution of the test blood until it matches a standard are less accurate and are now seldom used.

Compounds and standards

Oxyhaemoglobin

Oxyhaemoglobin is the simplest compound to use and can be prepared by dilution of blood, usually 1 in 200, in very dilute ammonia. Standards of this compound will not keep and so artificial standards are used. A grey solution (Thompson, 1946) or grey screen calibrated to absorb the same amount of light as a known concentration of oxyhaemoglobin can be used. The amount of light absorbed by this compound can be measured either

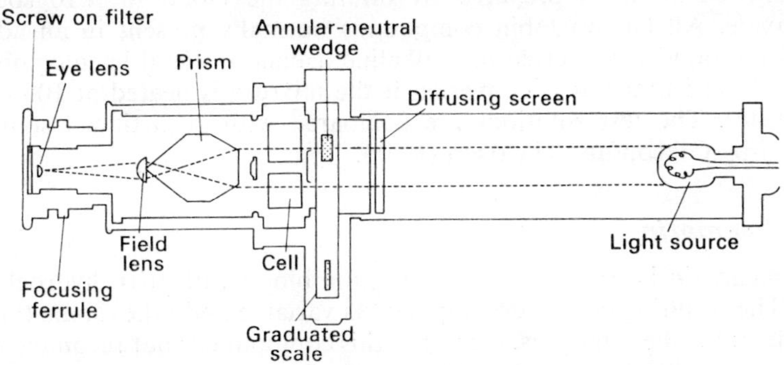

Fig. 1.2. MRC grey-wedge photometer used for haemoglobin estimation.

in a photo-electric absorptionometer or in the MRC grey-wedge photometer. Because most haemoglobin compounds absorb a similar quantity of light as oxyhaemoglobin, this method measures the total haemoglobin pigments present.

Cyanmethaemoglobin

Cyanmethaemoglobin (haemoglobincyanide) is the most stable compound in general use; standards of the compound itself keep for several months. It is prepared by diluting blood in a solution containing sodium bicarbonate, potassium cyanide and potassium ferricyanide. A theoretical disadvantage is that cyanide is used. Another disadvantage is that the solution has to be left for 3 minutes before being read, but this has been overcome in automated machines. The use of the pigment is becoming increasingly popular and an International Standard is available.

Carboxyhaemoglobin

Carboxyhaemoglobin, which is prepared by bubbling coal gas or carbon monoxide through a dilution of blood in 0·04% ammonia, has been widely used in the past. A disadvantage of using this compound is the necessity of having a source of gas. Because any methaemoglobin or sulphaemoglobin present is not converted into carboxyhaemoglobin, interference may occur in the comparison of the test and standard. Advantages are that its standards are reasonably stable and a colour standard has been defined by the British Standards Institution.

Alkaline haematin

Alkaline haematin is prepared by diluting the blood in N/10 sodium hydroxide. All haemoglobin compounds normally present in an adult's blood are rapidly converted into alkaline haematin. Fetal haemoglobin is relatively resistant but is converted if the mixture is heated at 100°C for 5 minutes. The test solutions are compared with an artificial standard devised by Gibson and Harrison (1945).

Acid haematin

Acid haematin is prepared by diluting the blood with N/10 hydrochloric acid. The resulting colour development is variable and takes some time to complete; for these reasons, the use of this compound is not recommended.

Screening methods

Measurements of the specific gravity of blood have been widely used as screening tests; for example, in the selection of blood donors. When a drop of blood is dropped on to a copper sulphate solution the proteins on its outside are denatured so that the drop becomes a compact sphere. If the specific gravity is greater than that of the solution it sinks, if less it floats. If the copper sulphate solution has a specific gravity of 1,053, all drops which sink can be accepted as containing more than 12 g/100 ml of haemoglobin. Plasma proteins also affect the specific gravity but only rarely will they be sufficiently abnormal to interfere with the test.

Patients whose blood floats should have their haemoglobin concentration estimated by one of the colorimetric methods.

Accuracy of haemoglobin estimations

Sampling errors both from the patient and from a container may affect the results of haemoglobin estimations. To these must be added the errors of pipettes and measuring instruments; also, human error may play a part. Generally speaking, the results recorded by a laboratory using a colorimetric method should have a 95% probability of being within 10% of the correct reading.

Normal haemoglobin values

Values accepted as normal in adults are 13·5–18 g/100 ml in men and 11·5–16·4 g/100 ml in women. It has been suggested that the sex difference is due to chronic iron deficiency in women, but, whilst it is true that the haemoglobin level of women can often be raised by iron therapy, most haematologists consider that there is a physiological difference. The haemoglobin level of newborn infants is very high, being in the range 18–28 g/100 ml; this drops to 10–15 g/100 ml by 6 months of age, remaining in this region until 10 years of age and then rising steadily to adult levels during adolescence (Fig. 1.3).

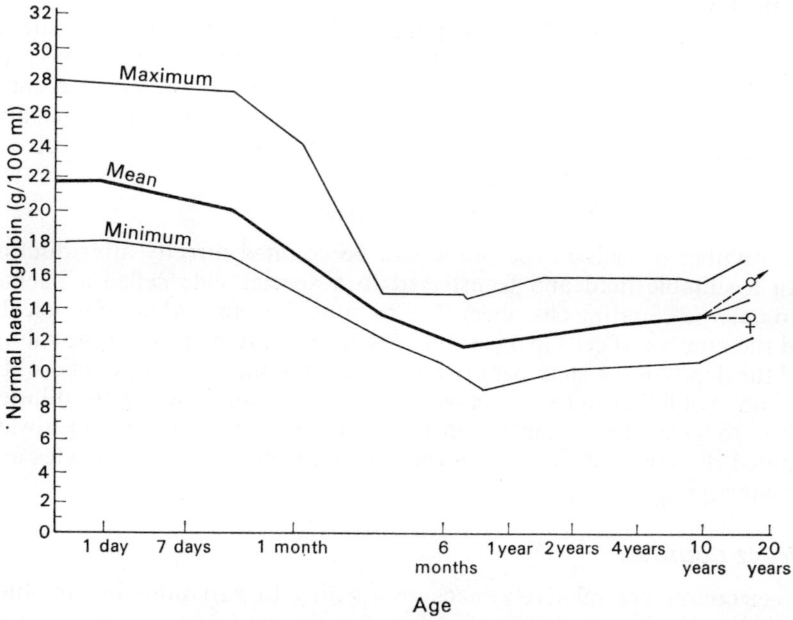

Fig. 1.3. Normal haemoglobin at different ages.

Further details of haemoglobin chemistry and metabolism and their disorders are given in Chapters 2 and 3.

Haematocrit

When blood containing a suitable anticoagulant is centrifuged, it separates into an upper plasma layer and a lower cellular layer. The volume of cells compared with that of the whole blood is expressed as a percentage and is called the packed cell volume (PCV). Usually the combined leucocytes and platelets, which are found as a 'buffy' coat above the erythrocytes, are less than 1% of the total value. If they form more, the result should be reported both as the erythrocyte cell volume and the leucocyte cell volume. The speed of centrifugation, time and the osmotic tonicity of the anticoagulant affect the results and should therefore be standardized.

Wintrobe's method was once in common use. Usually the ESR was first recorded, the tube then being placed on the centrifuge and spun at 3,000 r.p.m. for 30 minutes. Normal values are 40–52% for men and 35–47% for women. At birth the volume may be as high as 60%, dropping to 32–44% at the age of 1 year, remaining in this range until 10 years and then rising to adult levels during adolescence. This examination is accurate to within 1–2%.

A micro-method employing capillary tubes which are spun in a special centrifuge for 5 minutes is helpful when only small volumes of blood are available and is used as the routine method in many laboratories. Recently, electronic methods have been developed and one automated machine actually calculates the value from the size and number of the red cells.

Cell counts

The number of cells in the blood can be counted directly after dilution with a suitable fluid and transferred to a special slide called a haemocytometer (a counting chamber). The chamber is examined microscopically and the number of cells in a certain area counted. As the size of the rulings and the depth of the chamber are known, the number of cells per microlitre (μl; mm^3) of fluid can be calculated. This figure is multiplied by the dilution factor to give the concentration in the blood. Erythrocytes are always counted directly and this is also the preferred method for leucocytes and thrombocytes.

Direct counts

Direct counts are relatively inaccurate owing to variations in sampling, pipetting, distribution in the chamber and observer error. Errors of up to 20% are not uncommon. In recent years electronic cell counters have been introduced; they are generally more accurate than the older methods and are less laborious. However, each machine must be considered and evaluated separately as they are subject to individual errors.

Indirect counts

Indirect counts can be made by counting the proportion of unknown cells in a film to that of cells already counted directly. The absolute concentration can then be calculated by multiplying the proportion by the known cell count. This principle is employed in the differential leucocyte count, using the total leucocyte count as a standard. Reticulocytes and platelets can also be counted in this way, using the total red cell count as the standard. Indirect cell counts are less accurate than direct counts since further distribution and observer errors occur.

Erythrocyte counts

Total direct erythrocyte counts are usually performed by counting the number of cells in the haemocytometer after diluting the blood 1 in 200. Red cells can also be counted on an electronic counter after dilution by 1 in 50,000. The normal range for erythrocyte count is $4{\cdot}5$–$6{\cdot}5 \times 10^6/\mu l$ in males, and $3{\cdot}9$–$5{\cdot}6 \times 10^6/\mu l$ in females. At birth the count is considerably higher.

Red cell indices

Mean cell haemoglobin concentration (MCHC)

The haemoglobin concentration of red cells can be expressed as a percentage and called the MCHC. It can be calculated by determining the number of grammes of haemoglobin in 100 ml of red cells.

If the haemoglobin content of the blood is x grammes in 100 ml and the packed cell volume (PCV) is y, then there are x grammes of haemoglobin in y ml of erythrocytes.

The formula is usually written:

$$\text{MCHC} = \frac{\text{Hb in grammes per 100 ml blood}}{\text{PCV}\,\%} \times 100\,\%$$

For example, if the haemoglobin is 14 g/100 ml and the PCV is 40%, then the MCHC = 1,400/40 = 35%. Normal values are 32–36%. This measurement is relatively accurate, being based on the PCV which has a 1–2% error and on the haemoglobin concentration which has a 10% error. Automated electronic counters calculate the MCHC in different ways and this will affect the values obtained.

Mean cell volume (MCV)

The average volume of the erythrocyte is obtained by dividing the volume of erythrocytes by their numbers in any given volume of blood. If the PCV is $y\%$ and the erythrocyte count $z \times 10^6/\mu l$, then in 1 litre of blood the volume of cells will be $10y$ ml and the number of cells $z10^6 \times 10^6 = z10^{12}$ (since there are 10^6 μl in each litre).

The average volume of each cell is therefore $10y/z10^{12}$ ml. Since 1 ml = 10^{12} femtolitres (fl), the average cell volume will be

$$\frac{10y}{z10^{12}} \times 10^{12} \text{ or } \frac{10y}{z} \text{ fl}$$

The formula is usually written as:

$$\text{MCV, in fl} = \frac{\text{PCV} \times 10}{\text{RBC, in millions, per } \mu l}$$

For example, if PCV = 45 and RBC = 5, then MCV = $(45 \times 10)/5$ = 90 fl. The normal values are 76–96 fl. This index depends upon the erythrocyte count and is therefore relatively inaccurate unless the latter is determined electronically.

Mean cell haemoglobin (*MCH*)

This is a measure of the average haemoglobin content of each cell and is obtained by dividing the amount of haemoglobin by the number of red cells in any given unit of blood.

If the haemoglobin content is x g/100 ml and the erythrocyte count $y\ 10^6/\mu l$, then in 1 litre of blood there are $10x$ g of haemoglobin and $y\ 10^{12}$ erythrocytes. The average haemoglobin content of each erythrocyte is therefore $x10/y10^{12}$ of Hb. As 1 g = 10^{12} picogrammes (pg; micromicrogrammes) the average cell haemoglobin is:

$$\frac{10x}{y10^{12}} \times 10^{12} = \frac{10x}{y}\ \text{pg}$$

The formula is usually written:

$$\text{MCH, in pg} = \frac{\text{haemoglobin, in g, per 100 ml} \times 10}{\text{erythrocytes, in millions, per } \mu l}$$

The normal values are 27–32 pg. This index again depends upon the erythrocyte count and is therefore relatively inaccurate.

Erythrocyte mean cell diameter

Another measurement which is sometimes made is the erythrocyte mean cell diameter; all methods are laborious and are therefore used more often in research than in routine studies. They depend upon the measurement of the diameter of at least 100 red cells in a stained blood film either by microscopy using an eyepiece micrometer or after projection on to a suitable screen and measuring the image. The cells are classified into groups differing by 0·5 μm. In adults the majority of cells fall into the range 6·5–8 μm (mean 7·2 μm), with the occasional larger or smaller cell. The diameter is greater (8–9 μm) at birth, dropping to 5 μm at 3 months and rising again to 7 μm by 1 year. If the diameters are plotted on an abscissa and the frequencies on the ordinate, a size distribution (Price-Jones) curve is obtained.

The mean cell diameter can be measured more quickly by diffraction methods; however, this does not give any idea of the frequencies of different diameters and usually a careful observation of a well-stained blood film suffices. Using electronic counters incorporating pulse height analysis and read-out, a red cell volume distribution curve which corresponds to the Price-Jones curve can be obtained automatically.

Reticulocyte counts

Reticulocytes are usually counted indirectly after vital staining with cresyl blue. The number of reticulocytes per 100 red cells is expressed as a percentage. Absolute figures are not usually given. The normal range is from 0·2 to 2%.

Leucocyte counts

Total direct counts

The total leucocyte count is usually measured in the haemocytometer after dilution of the whole blood 1 in 20 with a special fluid which lyses the red cells. Electronic counters can also be used. The normal adult range is 4,000–10,000/μl. In children the count is higher, being 10,000–25,000/μl at birth, dropping to 5,000–12,500/μl at the age of 10 years and followed by a further drop to the adult level by the age of 20 years.

Differential counts

These are made by classifying at least 100 leucocytes on the blood film. The total count is then multiplied by the proportion present to give the absolute numbers present. The normal ranges for the numbers of the different types of leucocytes in the adult are: neutrophils, 2,500–7,500/μl; lymphocytes, 1,500–3,500/μl; monocytes, 200–800/μl; eosinophils, 40–400/μl; basophils, 15–100/μl. In children there are relatively more lymphocytes which often outnumber the neutrophils.

Direct eosinophil counts

Such counts are sometimes performed by counting cells in a haemocytometer after dilution of the blood with a special diluting fluid.

Thrombocyte counts

Thrombocytes are usually counted directly in a haemocytometer after dilution of the blood 1 in 100. A variety of special fluids are used, some of which will lyse the red cells. Experience is required to obtain reliable results; values vary somewhat according to the method used, but 150,000–400,000/μl can be accepted as normal. Indirect counts can be made by counting the number of platelets in each of ten microscopical fields, each containing approximately 100 red cells. This gives the numbers per thousand red cells. Multiplication by the red cell count in millions therefore gives the number of platelets in thousands per microlitre. This method is relatively inaccurate but is of some value in practice.

Erythrocyte sedimentation rate

When blood containing an anticoagulant is allowed to stand, the erythrocytes aggregate to form cylinders of cells, called rouleaux. The rate at which this occurs is called the erythrocyte sedimentation rate (ESR). The factors involved are complex; most important are the rate at which rouleaux form and their size, and these in turn are dependent on the plasma fibrinogen and globulins and possibly upon protein released into the plasma during inflammatory reactions (agglomerins). The haemoglobin concentration, dilution of the blood, length and diameters of the tubes used in the test and temperatures are important and must be standardized.

The rate is generally increased in diseases in which tissue destruction occurs and its measurement is of value in assessing both the severity of such diseases and the progress of a patient. Two methods are in common use.

Westergren's method

Westergren's method is the more sensitive. Four volumes of blood, which must be freshly drawn, are mixed with one volume of 3·8 % sodium citrate solution. After mixing, the blood is drawn up into a tube 2 mm in diameter and 200 mm long, which is fixed in a special rack which holds it vertically and seals the bottom end. The rate of erythrocyte sedimentation after 1 hour is measured; the normal fall is 0–20 mm. Blood collected into solid oxalate or EDTA can be used for the test provided it has not been collected for more than a few hours and is diluted with the appropriate volume of citrate solution.

Wintrobe's method

Wintrobe's method had the advantage that the same tubes could be used for PCV determination. Blood collected into solid anticoagulants is usually used (the oxalate mixture of Heller and Paul was used by Wintrobe, but many laboratories now use EDTA). After mixing, a portion of the blood is transferred to a tube 2 mm in diameter and 100 mm in length, which is sealed at the bottom end. The tube is placed in a special rack which holds it vertically and the fall of erythrocyte sedimentation after 1 hour is measured. The normal drop is 3–7 mm. This method is less sensitive than the Westergren because the blood is not diluted and the red cells have less distance in which to sediment before packing slows their rate of fall.

Recently, measurements of plasma viscosity have been introduced; like the ESR, they depend on changes in plasma proteins but are unaffected by factors acting through the red cells.

Blood films

In preparing blood for microscopy a small drop is first spread on a glass slide and allowed to dry. Considerable care and practice are required to obtain a good film; details are given in the practical manuals. After drying, the cells are fixed and stained. Methanol is usually used as the fixative and is followed by staining with one of the Romanowsky stains. These stains are prepared from mixtures of methylene blue and eosin by methods which involve the production of purple dyes (azures) which are oxidation products of methylene blue. Leishman's stain is commonly used in Britain, and Wright's stain in the U.S.A.

Another technique, the Pappenheim panoptic method, involves the use of two stains. After fixation, films are first stained with May–Grunwald's or Jenner's stain, which are simple methylene blue–eosin preparations. The films are then counterstained with diluted Giemsa stain, which is a purified azure preparation. Only reliable grades of stain should be used. The results obtained are generally similar, but slight variation may occur with the different types of stain, with the pH of the buffer used in diluting and with the thickness of the blood films. Structures which stain red are called acidophilic (syn. eosinophilic) and are probably alkaline in reaction; those which stain blue are basophilic and probably are acid in reaction. All shades between red and blue may be seen. Structures which stain purple are often described as being azurophilic and are best seen after Giemsa staining.

Examination of the stained film

The film should first be examined under the lower power of the microscope to see if it is suitably stained. The relative numbers of red and white cells are assessed and a suitable area is chosen for higher power examination. Oil immersion microscopy may be needed to see the finer cellular details (Plate 1, facing p. 24).

Erythrocytes

The erythrocytes are seen as non-nucleated round discs about 7μm in diameter. The cell stains red, but the centre of the cell is less densely stained than the periphery. This is because the erythrocyte is a biconcave disc and is thinner in the middle than at the edges. In young erythrocytes the cytoplasm has a bluish hue. Such cells, which form 0·5–2% of the erythrocytes, are said to be polychromatic. Abnormalities of erythrocyte morphology and staining are described later in this chapter.

Leucocytes

The white cells can be divided into the three series—granulocytes, lymphocytes and monocytes—by their appearances in the panoptic-stained films. Granulocytes are further subdivided into three types—neutrophils, eosinophils and basophils—depending upon the nature of the granules in their cytoplasm.

Neutrophil granulocytes

Neutrophil granulocytes are usually the leucocytes seen most frequently in smears of normal adult blood. They are 10–14 μm in diameter. The nucleus, which stains deep violet, may be of various shapes and gives rise to the alternative name of neutrophil polymorphonuclear leucocyte (abbreviated to polymorph). In the young form (juvenile neutrophil, stab, staff or band cell) the nucleus, which is not segmented, appears tubular and is bent into a variety of shapes of which the C and Z are typical. In the older forms (segmented neutrophils) the nucleus is divided into two to five lobes which are connected by a fine chromatin bridge. In females, some of the neutrophil nuclei have an additional small lobe known as a drumstick. This feature can be used to 'sex' blood films but experience is needed in the identification of true drumsticks and in the interpretation of results. The cytoplasm of the neutrophils stains a light pink colour and contains granules which are stained red to violet and are usually small but vary somewhat in size and number. Sometimes none can be seen; occasionally they are very prominent and are then called 'toxic granules'.

Eosinophil granulocytes

Eosinophil granulocytes generally resemble neutrophils, but are slightly larger. The nucleus usually contains two lobes and the cytoplasm is crowded with relatively large reddish-brown granules.

Basophil granulocytes

Basophil granulocytes generally resemble neutrophils. The nucleus is often obscured by large violet granules which fill the cytoplasm.

Lymphocytes

Lymphocytes are the smallest leucocytes in the blood, varying from about 7 to 14 μm in diameter; two types are sometimes distinguished, the small and the large. The nucleus is rounded or slightly indented and fills most of the cell. The nuclear material is arranged in dense masses which stain a very deep purple. The cytoplasm is a clear light blue and sometimes contains a few azurophilic granules.

Monocytes

Monocytes are the largest leucocytes in the blood; they vary from about 15 to 25 μm in diameter. The nucleus is typically slightly indented into two or three lobes, but may be of various other shapes. It has an open chromatin network and is slightly purple in colour. The cytoplasm is a hazy light blue and usually contains a few granules. The cell is often irregular in shape.

Abnormal leucocytes are described later.

Thrombocytes

Thrombocytes (platelets) are seen in panoptic-stained films as small (2–5 μm in diameter) non-nucleated round or oval cells. The cytoplasm contains reddish-purple granules in the centre with a clear zone at the edges. Clumps of thrombocytes are often found in blood smears. Abnormal forms are described later.

Bone marrow examination

Marrow can usually be aspirated from a bone with comparative ease and the haemopoietic cells examined. Less commonly it is necessary to examine histologically a portion of marrow; in this case a small portion of spongy bone has to be removed by trephine biopsy.

Aspiration biopsy

In adults active haemopoietic marrow is present in the flat bones and aspiration specimens are most frequently taken from the sternum, ilium and vertebral spines. In infants the upper end of the tibia is often used, and in children the ilium or vertebral spines. The skin and soft tissue over the puncture site are anaesthetized with a local anaesthetic and a special marrow puncture needle is inserted through the outer cortex of the bone. Bone marrow is then sucked into the syringe, transferred to glass slides and smeared. Some haematologists also pick out flecks of marrow with forceps and then squash them on to glass slides. Aspirate may also be allowed to clot in a small tube for histological examination. A variety of needles and techniques are used and are described in detail in practical manuals. Normal cells seen in films made from bone marrow and stained by panoptic method are described below (Plate 1, facing p. 24).

Trephine biopsy

In some patients it is not possible to aspirate bone marrow and in others it is desirable to see the histological structure of the spongy bone. This can be achieved by a trephine biopsy. Special trephine needles are available which allow a small core of bone 2–4·5 mm in diameter and 10–20 mm in length to be cored from the ilium. Imprints on to glass slides may be made from the ends of such cores. The core then is submitted for histological sectioning and examination.

Normal morphology of bone marrow cells

The parent cell from which the other haemopoietic cells are derived is called the haemocytoblast (Plate 1, facing p. 24). It is a large cell about 20 μm in diameter. The nucleus is primitive, having an open chromatin network and containing several nucleoli. These are the light blue areas in the nuclei which contain ribonucleoprotein (RNA protein) in contrast to the chromatin which is deoxyribonucleoprotein (DNA protein). This cell is thought to give rise to the other cell types.

Erythrocytic series

The most primitive cell recognizable in the erythroid series is the proerythroblast (pronormoblast). The cell is similar to, but slightly smaller than, the haemocytoblast; the cytoplasm is a shade deeper blue and the nuclear chromatin slightly more coarse. The next cell, the normoblast, is more easily recognized. The nuclear pattern is coarser and the cytoplasm less blue than that of the proerythroblast. During maturation there is a progressive condensation with the shrinkage of the nucleus and a loss of cytoplasmic basophilia. The early normoblast (normoblast A) still has a blue cytoplasm and for this reason is sometimes called the basophilic normoblast. The next cell, the intermediate normoblast (normoblast B), has a bluish-red cytoplasm due to the staining of both the remaining RNA and the developing haemoglobin. Finally, in the late normoblast (normoblast C) the cytoplasm is more red but retains a slight basophilia; the nucleus is very small and dark (pyknotic). The nucleus dissolves or is extruded, giving rise to a mature erythrocyte. In many cells polychromasia of the cytoplasm remains after loss of the nucleus. These are the polychromatic erythrocytes. In the vital cresyl blue preparation the cytoplasmic RNA of these cells shows up a network of blue-stained fibres and the cell is then called a reticulocyte.

Granulocytic series

The most primitive cell recognizable as a granulocyte is the myeloblast; it resembles the haemocytoblast but is a little smaller. Next in development is the promyelocyte which is generally similar, but with some azurophilic granules in the cytoplasm. Nucleoli or their remnants are still present and the cytoplasm is still blue. The blueness of the cytoplasm gradually decreases and the proportion of cytoplasm to nucleus increases as the cell matures. The next stage, the myelocyte, includes three different types depending upon the nature of the granules it contains. The neutrophils have granules which appear slightly reddish. The eosinophil has large and more markedly red granules and the basophil has large basophilic granules. The nucleus is oval or kidney-shaped. Myelocytes mature into metamyelocytes which have a horseshoe-shaped nucleus and these in turn give rise to the juvenile (non-segmented) granulocytes found in the peripheral blood. Subsequent lobulation of the nucleus gives rise to the segmented granulocytes.

Thrombocytic series

Thrombocytes develop by budding from megakaryocytes. Mature megakaryocytes are very large and are easy to find in the marrow specimens. The earlier stages are not so easily recognized. The megakaryoblast derived from the haemocytoblast undergoes polyploidy and then cytoplasmic granulation to become the mature platelet-producing megakaryocyte.

Lymphocytic series

Lymphocytes are formed in the lymphatic tissues by maturation of lymphoblasts. Lymphoblasts are not usually found in bone marrow aspirates, but lymphocytes may be present in variable numbers and some haematologists believe they can give rise to other cell types in the bone marrow.

Monocytic series

Monocytes are formed in the reticuloendothelial tissues throughout the body, including the bone marrow. They are probably formed in various ways, including maturation from the haemocytoblast through monoblast and promonocyte stages.

Other cells

Reticuloendothelial cells, plasma cells, tissue mast cells, osteoblasts and osteoclasts may be seen in the bone marrow aspirates. Cells foreign to the bone marrow and cells whose origin cannot be determined are also sometimes found. Although competent haematologists can recognize most cells in the bone marrow, some cells bearing features of more than one series sometimes make identification difficult. Furthermore, two authorities may classify a particular cell differently. Competence usually comes with experience and the novice should not be discouraged if he cannot classify all the cells found in normal marrow.

Examination of other haemopoietic tissues

Lymph node

Cells can be aspirated with ease from enlarged lymph nodes but their examination is rarely of diagnostic value. More commonly nodes are removed surgically and examined histologically. Inguinal nodes should be avoided if possible, and a 1–2 cm node removed from the axilla or neck.

Spleen

Aspiration biopsy of the spleen can provide adequate material for diagnosis in some disorders associated with splenomegaly. Histological examination of spleens removed at operation may also sometimes reveal a previously unsuspected disorder.

Liver

Histological section of liver needle biopsies are occasionally of value in haematological diseases.

Recommended supplementary reading

Textbooks

BRITTON, C. J. C. (1969). *Disorders of the Blood*, 10th ed. Churchill Livingstone, Edinburgh and London.
DE GRUCHY, G. C. (1970). *Clinical Haematology in Medical Practice*, 3rd ed. Blackwell, Oxford.
WINTROBE, M. M. (1967). *Clinical Haematology*, 6th ed. Kimpton, London.

Practical manuals

DACIE, J. V. and LEWIS, S. M. (1968). *Practical Haematology*, 4th ed. Churchill Livingstone, Edinburgh and London.
DARMADY, E. M. and DAVENPORT, S. G. T. (1963). *Haematological Technique*, 3rd ed. Churchill Livingstone, Edinburgh and London.
DELANEY, J. W. and GARRATTY, G. (1969). *Handbook of Haematological and Blood Transfusion Technique*, 2nd ed. Butterworths, London.

Haematology atlases

HAYHOE, F. G. J. and FLEMENS, R. J. (1969). *An Atlas of Haematological Cytology*. Wolfe, London.
ISRAELS, M. C. G. (1948). *An Atlas of Bone Marrow Pathology*, 4th ed. Heinemann Medical, London.
MCDONALD, G. A., DODDS, T. C. and CRUICKSHANK, B. (1970). *Atlas of Haematology*, 3rd ed. Churchill Livingstone, Edinburgh and London.
Sandoz Atlas of Haematology (1952). Sandoz, Basle.

Nuclear sexing of polymorphs

BARR, M. L. (1960). Cytological tests of chromosomal sex. In: *Recent Advances in Clinical Pathology*, Series III. Ed. S. C. Dyke. Churchill Livingstone, Edinburgh and London.

Haemoglobin estimation

GIBSON, Q. H. and HARRISON, D. C. (1945). An artificial standard for use in the estimation of haemoglobin. *Biochem. J.* **39**, 490.

KING, K. J. and WOOTTON, I. D. P. (1956). *Micro analysis in Medical Biochemistry*, 3rd ed. Churchill Livingstone, Edinburgh and London.

ONESTI, P., STENHOUSE, N. S. and WOODLIFF, H. J. (1969). A comparison of three simple haemoglobinometers. *Med. J. Aust.* **1**, 683–4.

THOMPSON, L. C. (1946). An inorganic grey solution. *Trans. Faraday Soc.* **42**, 663.

2 Erythropoiesis and its disorders

Introduction

Normal erythrocytes are produced in the bone marrow by the maturation of late normoblasts which, in their turn, are derived from earlier cells. A model for this process has been proposed by Lajtha in which each stem cell gives rise to 20 erythrocytes by various processes of multiplication and maturation (Fig. 2.1). This takes about 6 days from stem cell to the reticulocyte and a further 5 days, part of which may be in the circulation, for final maturation to the erythrocyte. During this process about 10% of the precursor cells are destroyed. This waste is called ineffective erythropoiesis.

Erythropoiesis is controlled by the hormone erythropoietin. Tissue anoxia leads to the increased production of renal erythropoietic factor or erythrogenin by the kidney and this acts on an α_1-globulin plasma substrate to form erythropoietin. This then acts on those stem cells committed for erythropoiesis and also on the later nucleated erythroid precursors to increase their rate of production. The nutrients necessary for erythropoiesis include proteins, vitamins (folate, cobalamin, ascorbic acid, pyridoxine, riboflavine, pantothenic acid and nicotinic acid) and minerals (iron, cobalt and copper).

Some $2{\cdot}1 \times 10^{11}$ erythrocytes leave the bone marrow each day and survive for about 120 days in the circulation. Thus the blood has a turnover rate of about 0·8% per day. Old erythrocytes are removed from the circulation by the cells of the reticuloendothelial system. Their proteins are broken down to amino acids which may be reutilized or deaminated. The iron released is taken up by the body stores or used for new haemoglobin synthesis and the pigment portion of the haem is excreted in the bile as bilirubin.

Normal red cell production and destruction are carefully balanced and, in disease, disturbance may take place in either. They may be due to intrinsic defects of erythropoiesis or to extrinsic causes. Associated with these disorders there may be abnormality of erythrocyte mass, numbers, morphology, staining, osmotic and mechanical fragility, life span and biochemistry. These are considered in the following section.

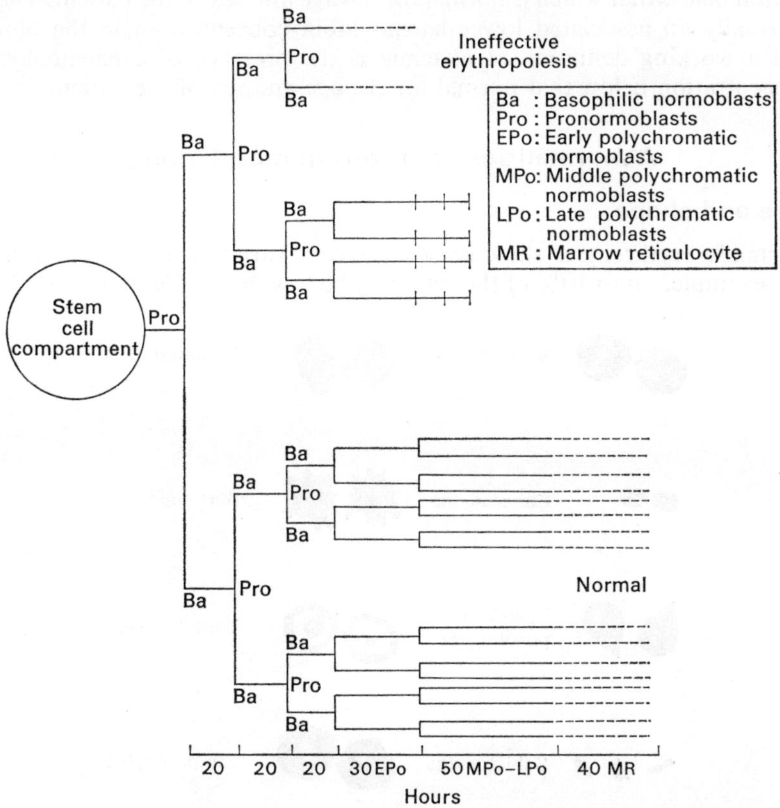

Fig. 2.1. Kinetic model of erythroid maturation (adapted from Lajtha).

Key **Ba:** Basophilic normoblasts
Pro: Pronormoblasts
E Po: Early polychromatic normoblasts
M Po: Middle polychromatic normoblasts
LPo: Late polychromatic normoblasts
MR: Marrow reticulocyte

ERYTHROCYTE ABNORMALITIES

Abnormalities of erythrocyte mass and numbers

The presence of too few or defective erythrocytes in the body is called anaemia. It may be due to poor production of red cells by the bone marrow, to excessive losses or to a combination of the two. The body red cell mass can be measured by tagging a known amount of cells with radiochromium and then measuring the dilution of radioactivity when these cells are injected. Normal values are 26–33 ml of red cells per kg in males and

19–29 ml/kg in females. Provided there is no disturbance of the blood haematocrit the anaemia will usually be reflected in an erythrocyte concentration below that which is normal for the age and sex of the patient. There is usually an associated lower haemoglobin concentration in the blood and a working definition of anaemia is the presence of a haemoglobin concentration below that normal for the age and sex of the patient.

Abnormalities of erythroid morphology

Size and shape

Normally erythrocytes show some degree of variation in size (Fig. 2.2). For example, up to 10% of the cells may be less than 6·5 μm or more than

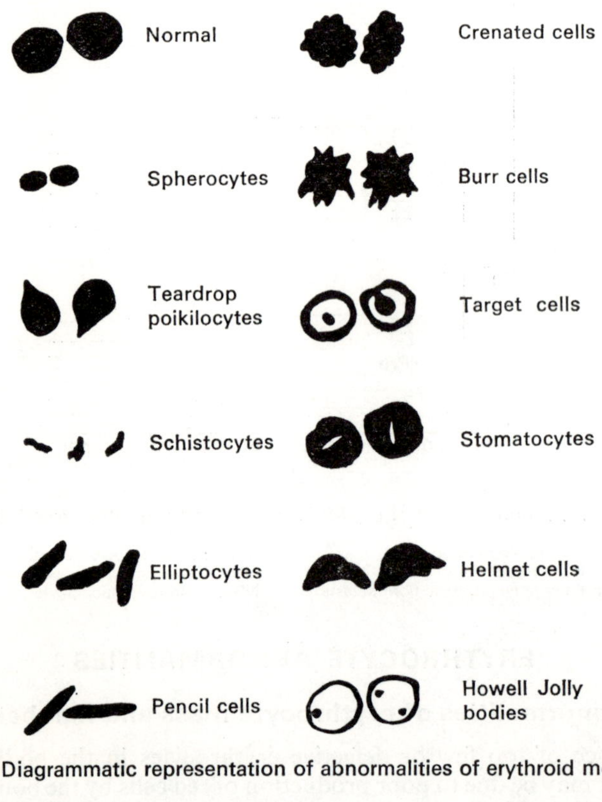

Fig. 2.2. Diagrammatic representation of abnormalities of erythroid morphology.

8 μm in diameter. If this variation in size is greater than normal, anisocytosis is said to be present. Cells smaller than 6·5 μm are called microcytes. Macrocytes are derived from either macronormoblasts or megaloblasts. Cells may also be thinner or thicker than normal. Thin cells, called lepto-

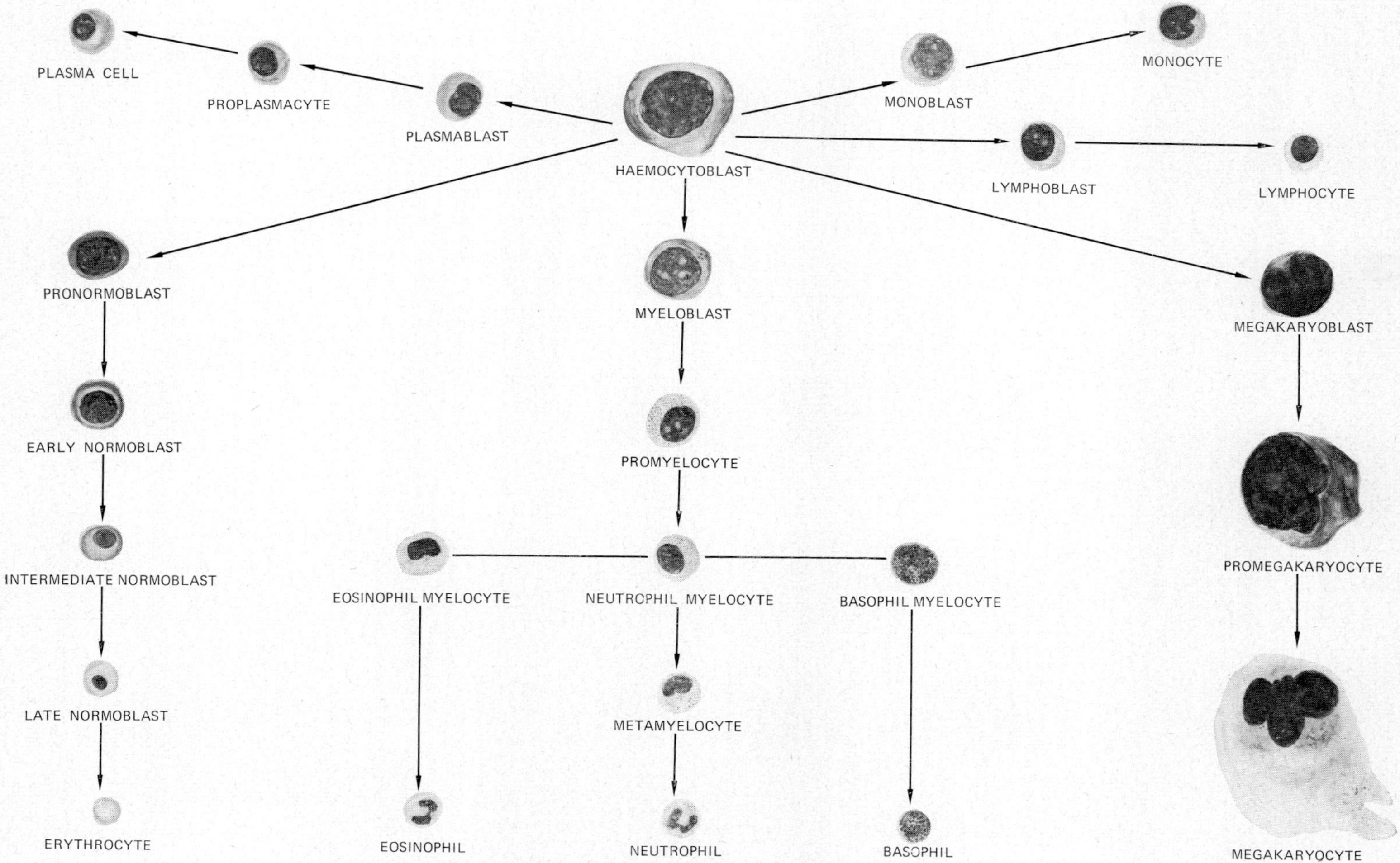

Plate 1. Normal morphology of blood and bone marrow cells.

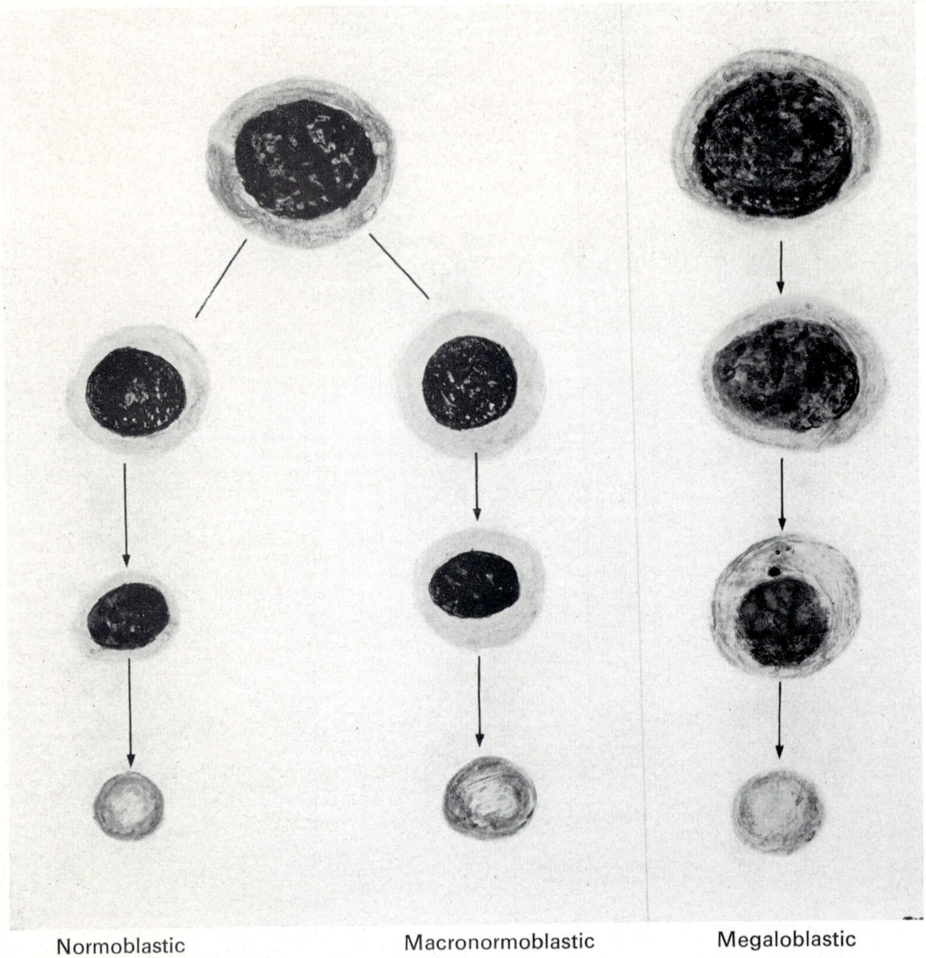

Normoblastic Macronormoblastic Megaloblastic

Plate 2. Diagrammatic illustration of the differences between normoblastic and megaloblastic maturation of erythroblasts.

cytes, are usually also large; they are relatively resistant to rupture by hypotonic saline. Thick cells usually have a small diameter; the result is a spherical cell called a microspherocyte which is relatively sensitive to rupture by hypotonic saline (see Fig. 2.4).

Irregularly shaped erythrocytes, many of which may be pear-shaped or likened to 'teardrops', are called poikilocytes; tiny fragments are sometimes called schistocytes. A small percentage of oval-shaped red cells, called ovalocytes, may be present in normal blood. The numbers may be moderately increased in various anaemias. More markedly oval-shaped cells, called elliptocytes, are found in hereditary elliptocytosis. Very thin elongated cells, called pencil cells, are seen in hypochromic anaemia.

Sickle and other peculiar shapes are found in erythrocytes containing reduced haemoglobin S (Chapter 3).

If erythrocytes are placed in hypertonic solutions they shrink and form prickles, and are then called crenated or burr cells, depending on the degree of shrinkage. They are sometimes present in the blood of patients with uraemia.

Staining

Pale cells which have a low content of haemoglobin are said to be hypochromic. In severe hypochromasia the cells may resemble a stained ring and may then be called anulocytes. Cells cannot be supersaturated with haemoglobin and so hyperchromasia does not exist. In the past the term has, however, been used in connection with normochromic macrocytes because they contain more than the average amount of haemoglobin. Microspherocytes stain darkly because of their increased thickness. Leptocytes which have a dark centre surrounded by a paler area with another dark ring on the outside are called target cells. Polychromatic cells normally form 1–2% of the erythrocytes; in active blood regeneration their numbers are increased. They have a bluish tinge and are slightly larger than older cells.

Inclusions

Cabot's rings are violet rings or figures of eight which are occasionally seen in erythrocytes. Howell–Jolly bodies are round violet dots about 1 μm in diameter and several may be seen in a single erythrocyte. Smaller finer particles called nuclear dust are occasionally found. These three types of material are all nuclear remnants; they are sometimes seen in anaemia and are especially common after splenectomy.

Erythrocytes showing basophilic stippling are occasionally seen in normal blood smears. Increased numbers are sometimes found in anaemia and are characteristically seen in lead poisoning and in thalassaemia.

Pappenheimer bodies are basophilic granules of varying size sometimes seen in erythrocytes. If the blood film is stained by the prussian blue technique the granules give a positive blue reaction for free iron, and the cells are called siderocytes. They are sometimes seen in anaemia and are especially common after splenectomy.

Heinz bodies are refractile globules seen in unstained erythrocytes or after supravital staining with methyl violet. They may be dissolved by panoptic stains and thus not be seen in the usual blood film. Heinz bodies are usually found only in patients suffering from some forms of haemolytic anaemia and after splenectomy. They are formed from oxidized, denatured haemoglobin.

Small vacuoles may be seen in the red cells of patients who have undergone splenectomy (post-splenectomy vacuoles).

Abnormalities of erythrocyte precursors

Macro- and micronormoblasts

Normoblasts which are larger than normal but which have a normal nuclear pattern are called macronormoblasts (see Plate 2, facing p. 25). They generally resemble normal normoblasts except for the relatively greater cytoplasmic nuclear ratio. They are usually seen when there is hyperplasia of the erythroid tissue following an increased demand for blood and are associated with a macrocytosis in the peripheral blood.

Micronormoblasts are smaller than normal. They generally resemble normal normoblasts but have relatively less cytoplasm, which has a ragged appearance and is hypochromic. They are found in iron-deficiency anaemia and are associated with microcytosis and hypochromasia in the peripheral blood.

Megaloblasts

An abnormal series of cells is formed in the bone marrow in cobalamin and folate deficiencies (see Plate 2). The promegaloblast resembles the pronormoblast, but is larger (16–25 μm) and contains relatively more cytoplasm. The nuclear chromatin is even finer than that of the pronormoblast and this feature distinguishes it from the promacronormoblast in which the chromatin is coarser. The early, intermediate and later megaloblasts differ from their normal counterparts in being larger, having a greater cytoplasmic nuclear ratio and in the chromatin pattern of the nucleus. This is always much finer than in the normal cells and clumps of chromatin that are found only in late cells.

A megaloblastic marrow is usually associated with anaemia and the presence of macrocytes in the peripheral blood.

Nucleated red cells and reticulocytes in the peripheral blood

Nucleated red cells are not normally found in the peripheral blood. They may be present in erythroid hyperplasia (e.g. in haemolytic anaemias and megaloblastic anaemias) or in disturbances of the bone marrow (e.g. leucoerythroblastic anaemias, leukaemias and erythraemias).

Up to 2% of the erythrocytes in the peripheral blood may be reticulocytes; the number may be increased during erythroid hyperplasia or in other disorders of the bone marrow.

Other erythrocyte abnormalities

Osmotic fragility (Fig. 2.3)

Erythrocytes vary in their ability to withstand lysis in hypotonic saline. Normally, haemolysis commences in 0·5% saline at 20°C and is complete in 0·3% saline with a median corpuscular fragility of 0·40–0·45%. Blood which commences lysis in a concentration higher than normal shows

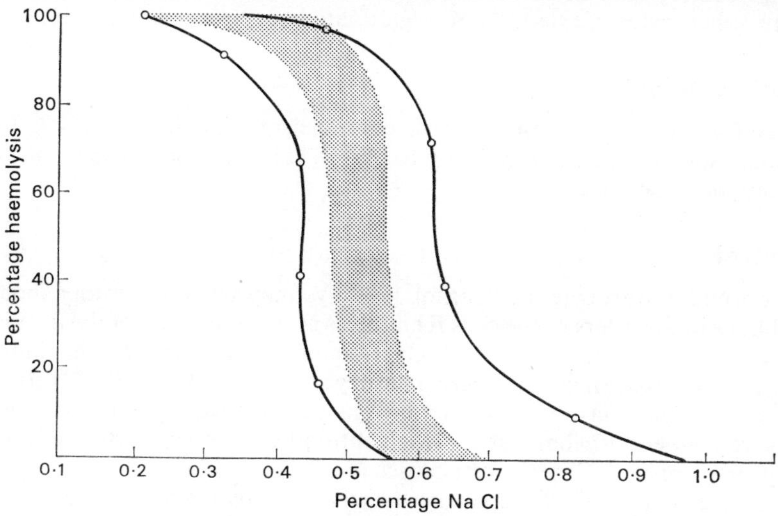

Fig. 2.3. Osmotic fragility curve of blood.

increased fragility (or decreased resistance to lysis). This blood usually contains microspherocytes and probably has been obtained from a patient with hereditary spherocytosis or acquired autoimmune haemolytic anaemia. Blood which is not completely lysed in saline concentrations of less than 0·3% shows decreased fragility (or increased resistance) and is found where leptocytes occur, as in iron deficiency anaemia, jaundice, sickle cell anaemia or thalassaemia.

The test is carried out under carefully standardized conditions of temperature and pH because these factors alter osmotic fragility. Results are recorded as the concentration of saline in which complete haemolysis occurs and median corpuscular fragility. It is usual to construct a fragility curve by plotting on graph paper the percentage of haemolysis in each tube for the corresponding saline concentration, using a range of hypotonic solutions (Fig 2.3).

Sometimes the osmotic fragility test is repeated after 24 hours' incubation at 37°C. This potentiates the increased fragility of erythrocytes in hereditary spherocytosis when compared with normals and may result in a normal curve becoming abnormal in mild hereditary spherocytosis. It is not specific since an increase has been found in certain non-spherocytic congenital haemolytic anaemias.

Mechanical fragility

Erythrocytes vary in their ability to withstand mechanical lysis. The test blood and control are shaken with glass beads for 1 hour. Normally there is 2–5% haemolysis. This is increased in some forms of haemolytic anaemia, where spherocytes, sickle cells or agglutinated corpuscles are present.

Autohaemolysis

Normal blood collected into a sterile container and incubated at 37°C for 24 hours shows little or no lysis (up to 0·5%). It is increased in some of the haemolytic anaemias.

Survival

The normal erythrocyte life span of 120 days may be considerably shortened both in disorders of the cells themselves and in disorders of the normal breakdown mechanism of the body. Abnormal erythrocytes having a shorter life span include microspherocytes and sickle cells. Normal erythrocytes may have a shortened life span as, for example, in disorders of the reticuloendothelial system, when antibodies to erythrocytes develop, in hypersplenism and in the reticuloses and leukaemias.

Measurements of the life span are usually made by tagging the cells with radioactive chromium. In this method some elution of the chromium occurs, giving a normal apparent half-life of about 26 days. (The half-life is that time at which 50% of the labelled cells are surviving.) Half-lives of less than 20 days indicate an appreciable degree of haemolysis.

BIOCHEMISTRY OF ERYTHROPOIESIS AND ITS DISORDERS

The production of biochemically normal red cells depends upon an adequate external environment of cofactors and metabolites and the presence in the precursor cells of the enzyme systems necessary for cellular synthesis and integrity. Defects may occur in either or may be combined. For the purpose of discussion it is convenient to divide the description of cellular biochemistry into nutritional requirements of erythropoiesis, haemoglobin metabolism, iron metabolism, haem metabolism, globin metabolism, haemoglobin variants, haemoglobin compounds and derivatives, and other aspects of erythrocyte biochemistry.

Nutritional requirements of erythropoiesis

The nutrients required for normal erythropoiesis include proteins, vitamins and minerals.

Proteins

Protein requirements are available to the erythroid tissues from the pool of amino acids normally present in the body. In mild protein malnutrition it is unusual for defective erythropoiesis to occur since the erythroid tissue appears to be able to take up amino acids preferentially. Severe deficiency or other associated deficiencies may be associated with anaemia.

Vitamins

The vitamins required include cobalamin, folate, ascorbic acid, pyridoxine, riboflavine, pantothenic acid and nicotinic acid.

The cobalamins

The cobalamins are converted in the body into enzyme cofactors necessary for normal erythropoiesis. In the absence of this factor megaloblastic anaemia and other metabolic disorders may occur.

Folates

Folates are converted into active forms in the body which are essential in the transfer of one carbon unit in a variety of metabolic pathways including nucleic acid synthesis. Their absence may lead to megaloblastic anaemia and other metabolic disorders. The relationship between the cobalamins and folates is discussed in Chapter 5.

Ascorbic acid

Ascorbic acid is thought to play a part in folic acid metabolism by helping in the production or maintenance of the reduced form. Very occasionally, deficiency results in a megaloblastic anaemia; more commonly, an associated iron deficiency anaemia is found.

Pyridoxine

Pyridoxine deficiency induced in laboratory rats causes anaemia and pyridoxine-responsive anaemias have been described in man. However, dietary deficiency is not the cause of such anaemias because they respond only to amounts of pyridoxine far in excess of normal physiological needs.

Riboflavine

Riboflavine is also needed by animals for normal erythropoiesis; human anaemias (probably of mixed aetiology) responding to this vitamin have been described.

Pantothenic acid and nicotinic acid

Pantothenic acid and nicotinic acid deficiency anaemias have been induced in laboratory animals. Anaemia due to a deficiency of, or responding to, these factors has not yet been described in man.

Minerals

The minerals necessary for erythropoiesis include iron, cobalt and copper. *Iron* deficiency is the commonest cause of anaemia. Its normal and disordered metabolism are discussed later. *Cobalt* deficiency anaemias are not seen in man but increased erythropoiesis due to excessive intake is occasionally found. *Copper* deficiency anaemias are not seen in man, but in animals deprivation of copper may lead to anaemia resembling that of iron deficiency. Copper is essential for haem synthesis because it is a component of the enzyme system catalysing the synthesis of porphobilinogen from δ-aminolaevulinic acid (ALA).

Haemoglobin metabolism

Introduction

Haemoglobin, the red pigment of the erythrocytes, consists of a closely related group of chromoproteins. Each molecule can be divided into four haem units and a globin moiety. The haem units contain iron and a tetrapyrrole structure and are the same, or very similar, in each type of haemoglobin. The globin part consists of two pairs of peptide chains, the amino acid constitution of which differs in each type of haemoglobin.

There are three normal adult haemoglobins—A, F and A_2—as well as many variants (Table 2.1).

Haem and globin are synthesized about the same time in the nucleated red cells. The exact sequence of their association in the cell is not known.

Haemoglobin catabolism takes place mainly in the cells of the reticular system, resulting in an iron-globin complex and in bilirubin production. A small amount of haemoglobin may be released into the plasma, giving a normal level of less than 5 mg/100 ml. In some disorders this is considerably increased. Haemoglobin in the plasma normally combines with a

Table 2.1

Haemoglobin	*Chains*	*Chemical change*
A	$\alpha_2^A\beta_2^A$	
A_2	$\alpha_2^A\delta$	
F	$\alpha_2^A\gamma$-	
C	$\alpha_2^A\beta_2^C$	Lysine for glutamyl
D	$\alpha_2^A\beta_2^O$	
G^1	$\alpha_2^A\beta_2^{G1}$	
H	β_4	
Q	$\alpha_2^Q\beta_2$	Valine
S	$\alpha_2^A\beta_2^S$	Valine for glutamyl
Barts	γ_4	

plasma α_2-mucoprotein called haptoglobin and the complex is then metabolized mainly in the liver but also in other reticular tissue. If this mechanism becomes saturated and haemoglobin released into the plasma reaches a concentration of about 100 mg/100 ml, then haemoglobinuria occurs, the haemoglobin may be taken up by the tubular epithelial cells of the kidney which become laden with iron and are subsequently desquamated into the urine where they can be detected by staining the urinary sediment by the prussian blue reaction (siderinuria). When large quantities of haemoglobin are released into the plasma some of the molecules break and the haem portion combines with albumin to form methaemalbumin; methaemoglobin may also be present in the plasma.

Further details of haemoglobin metabolism and its disorders follow under the headings of iron, haem and globin metabolism.

Iron metabolism

Iron is an essential constituent of the body, being a part of haemoglobin, myoglobin and the respiratory enzymes. It is also present in the body stores as ferritin and haemosiderin, and in the plasma as transferrin. Ferritin is water soluble, contains up to 40% by weight of ferric hydroxide and is not stained by the prussian blue reaction. Haemosiderin is granular, insoluble, contains up to 58% by weight of ferric hydroxide and gives a positive prussian blue reaction. Transferrin is a globulin, each molecule of which contains two iron atoms.

The total body iron of adults is between 3 and 5 g, of which about

1·5–3 g are in haemoglobin and 1–1·5 g in the body stores. The iron in myoglobin and various enzymes make up the balance (Fig. 2.4). A full-term infant has an initial supply of 0·3–0·5 g obtained from its mother; thereafter all iron must be obtained from food. Iron is not excreted as such, but 0·5–1 mg a day is lost in the bile and in desquamated cells. In women, an additional loss averaging 0·5–1 mg a day is usual due to menstruation.

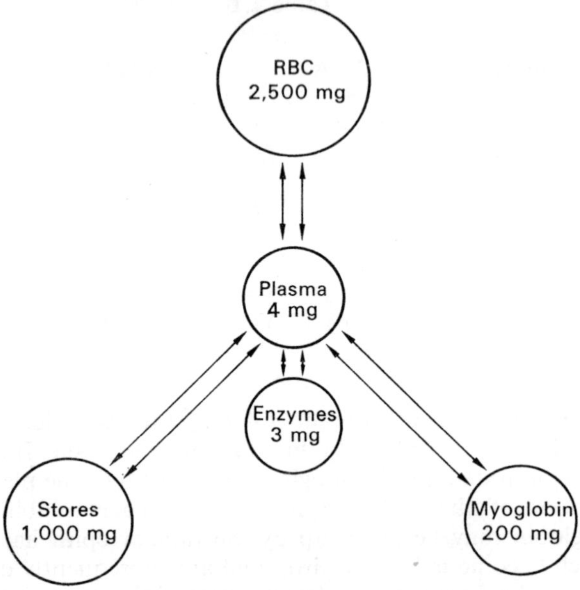

Fig. 2.4. Normal body iron distribution.

With pregnancy there is a loss of up to 1,200 mg but this is partially compensated by amenorrhoea. To make good these losses and to provide for growth, iron must be absorbed from the diet. Food contains various compounds of iron, but only those which can be converted into the ferrous form are readily absorbed.

A normal diet contains 10–15 mg of iron per day, but only about 5–10% of this is absorbed, giving a daily average intake of 0·5–1·5 mg. This is adequate for most men but may be inadequate for women who, in consequence, are commonly iron deficient.

Food rich in iron includes liver, kidney, egg yolk, meat, green vegetables and fruit. Milk contains only small quantities; a 'tea and toast' diet is poor in iron.

A variety of factors influence the absorption of iron. Ferrous iron is more readily absorbed than ferric and so reducing substances such as ascorbic acid favour absorption. Hydrochloric acid in the gastric juices also aids iron absorption. Active erythropoiesis and low iron stores in the body are associated with increased iron absorption and high iron stores, and decreased erythropoiesis with decreased absorption, although anaemia *per se* has been described as causing increased iron absorption. Exocrine secretions of the pancreas may be important in regulating dietary iron absorption. The amount of iron absorbed is also partially dependent upon

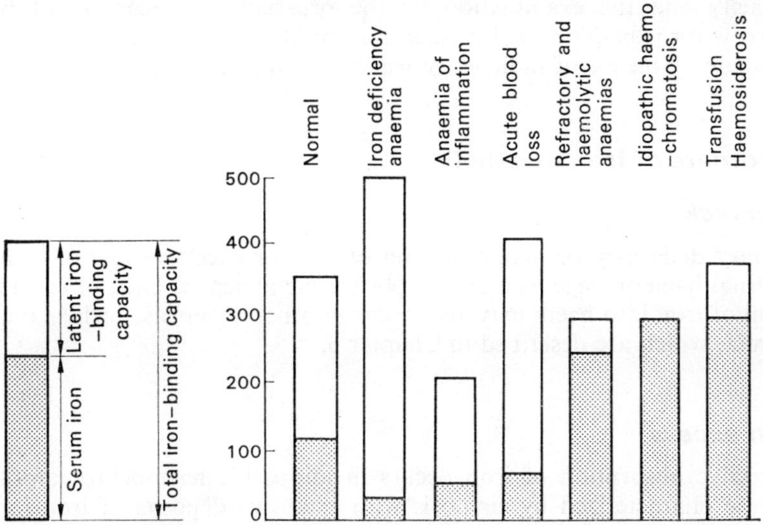

Fig. 2.5. Typical serum iron and total iron-binding capacity (transferrin) levels in various conditions. The serum levels are expressed in μg/100 ml.

the absolute amount available and, since there is no active excretion of iron, a mechanism controlling its absorption must be present. How this functions is not fully understood.

Iron is absorbed from the intestine in two phases; first a rapid phase from the lumen into the mucosa and, then, more slowly to the other tissues. The regulation and the form in which iron is transferred from the mucosal cells are not fully understood but are partly dependent on body iron stores. The iron, in due course, passes to the plasma where it is again oxidized to the ferric state and combines with a protein, transferrin (also called siderophillin or iron-binding protein). The iron in transferrin is deposited in the stores as ferritin or haemosiderin, or, after reduction, is used for haemoglobin synthesis. Some 25 mg of iron a day are used in haemoglobin synthesis, but most of this is provided by the breakdown of effete red cells. The plasma contains about 3 or 4 mg of iron, the concentration in plasma being 50–200 μg/100 ml. Normally the plasma iron-binding protein (transferrin) is only one-third saturated; when fully saturated, plasma can hold about 400 μg/100 ml of iron. Estimates of the serum iron and iron-binding capacity are of value in the diagnosis of some forms of anaemia (Fig. 2.5).

Methods of investigation

Iron deficiency in the body is reflected in a low haemoglobin concentration in the blood and in the individual red cells (low MCHC). Further investigations, which may be needed in the investigation of iron metabolism, include the measurement of the serum iron and the serum iron-binding capacity and the examination by the prussian blue reaction of bone marrow for iron deposits. Investigations of absorption and utilization can be made by means of radioactive tracer techniques.

Disorders of iron metabolism

Iron lack

Dietary deficiency or malabsorption of iron or excessive loss of iron by external haemorrhage lead to a hypochromic anaemia. Lack of incorporation of iron into haem may also occur in other anaemias, such as thalassaemia, which are described in Chapter 3.

Iron excess

Excessive absorption of iron occurs in idiopathic haemochromatosis, a disease characterized by cirrhosis with excessive deposits of iron in the liver, darkening of the skin and diabetes mellitus. Although the dietary intake of iron is normal, increased absorption occurs. The condition is inherited but the reasons for the increased absorption of iron are uncertain; a decreased concentration of an iron-binding protein normally present in gastric juice ('gastroferrin') is one suggestion.

Clinical features of haemochromatosis include hepatomegaly and disordered liver function due to the excessive iron deposits. If portal hypertension is present splenomegaly, ascites and oesophageal varices may develop. There may be loss of body hair, testicular atrophy and gynaecomastia, although gonadal hypofunction has been thought by some workers to be due to iron deposition in the pituitary or testes. Diabetes due to deposits in the pancreas is seen in 80% of patients, and increased skin pigmentation due to deposits of iron and melanin is almost universal.

The haemoglobin, leucocyte and platelet counts are usually normal unless there is bleeding or hypersplenism. The plasma iron is usually elevated and the iron-binding capacity completely or nearly completely saturated.

Liver biopsy usually provides conclusive evidence of iron overload plus accompanying cirrhosis. Bone marrow findings are rather unhelpful, the iron content being variable, though usually increased. Urinary iron excretion following an iron chelating agent may help in diagnosis since it is greatly elevated. Treatment is by repeated venesections; the iron chelating agents may have a place in therapy but the amount of iron removed in this way is small.

If excessive iron is deposited in the liver without causing fibrosis, the term haemosiderosis is used. This is usually found in patients with chronic anaemia following repeated blood transfusions or excessive parenteral iron therapy. A similar condition occurs in South African Bantus whose high liver iron content follows their habit of using iron pots for cooking and for brewing beer.

Haem metabolism

Haem synthesis and its disorders

Haem is ferroprotoporphyrin IX. Its synthesis is illustrated in Fig. 2.6.

Porphobilinogen is converted not only into uroporphyrinogen III but also to a lesser extent into uroporphyrinogen I. Derivatives of both these

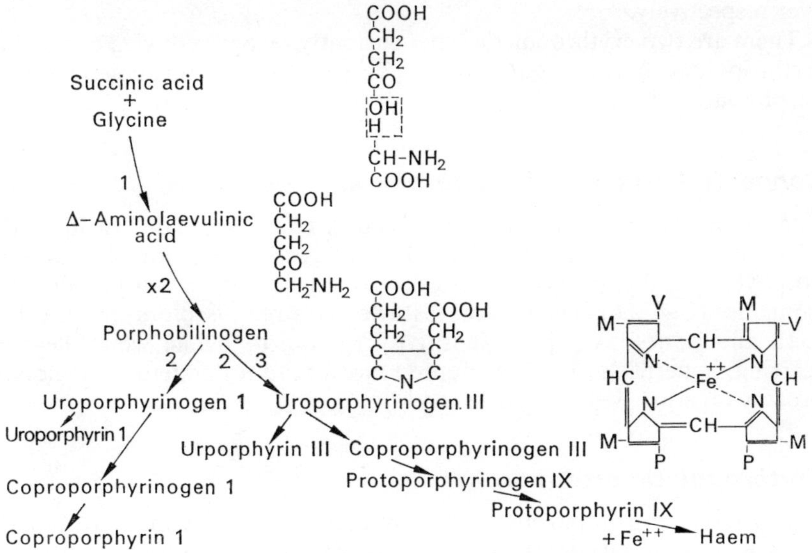

Fig. 2.6. The metabolic pathway of haem synthesis.

Key: (1) = Δ-ALA Synthetase; (2) = PBG Deaminase; (3) = PBG Isomerase; M = Methyl; P = Proprionyl; V = Vinyl

substances may be found in small quantities in the urine and the faeces as useless byproducts of haem synthesis.

Disorders of haem synthesis may be divided into two types: suppressive and abnormal.

Suppression

Suppression occurs in some anaemias such as thalassaemia or when there is a deficiency of precursors such as iron.

Abnormalities

Abnormalities of synthesis occur in the porphyrias and porphyrinurias. These conditions are characterized by an abnormal excretion of porphyrin compounds.

Porphyrias

The porphyrias are diseases both inherited and acquired where increased synthesis of porphyrins or porphyrin precursors occurs. They are best classified into two broad groups, erythropoietic and hepatic, indicating the origin of excess porphyrins to be the developing erythroid cell and the liver respectively.

There are two erythropoietic types currently recognized, viz., congenital erythropoietic porphyria (Gunther's disease) and erythropoietic protoporphyria.

Congenital erythropoietic porphyria

Congenital erythropoietic porphyria is an excessively rare disease inherited as an autosomal recessive and marked by gross overproduction of uroporphyrin I and coproporphyrin I due to a deficiency of porphobilinogen isomerase (Fig. 2.6). The clinical features are a red discoloration of urine, teeth and bones, skin photosensitivity leading to bullae which heal by scarring, hypertrichosis, pigmentation and a mild to moderate haemolytic process together with splenomegaly.

Erythropoietic protoporphyria

Erythropoietic protoporphyria is more common and its mode of inheritance is autosomal dominant. It, too, manifests photosensitivity but bullous formation is not a feature and scarring is much less of a problem. Urinary porphyrins are always normal and diagnosis is best made by the demonstration of an elevated erythrocyte protoporphyrin level in the absence of anaemia. Very large amounts of protoporphyrin are excreted in the faeces.

Porphyrias of hepatic origin can be considered in two groups: porphyria cutanea tarda and the hereditary acute porphyrias which are inherited as autosomal dominants.

Porphyria cutanea tarda

Porphyria cutanea tarda is generally thought to be an acquired disease, usually associated with alcoholic cirrhosis. The skin photosensitivity is similar to congenital erythropoietic porphyria. There is overproduction mainly of uroporphyrins. The drug hexachlorobenzene was the cause of an epidemic of porphyria in Turkey when it was added to bread as a fungicide. The disease was largely seen in children who became photosensitive, pigmented and developed hypertrichosis. The epidemic stopped upon withdrawal of the hexachlorobenzene.

Acute intermittent porphyria

Acute intermittent porphyria is not associated with cutaneous photosensitivity. The onset is frequently in the third decade with colicky abdominal pain, peripheral neuropathy or an organic brain syndrome. The abdominal pain is often accompanied by features suggesting small intestinal obstruction. During attacks there is often tachycardia and hypertension. The primary defect has been thought to be a failure of negative feedback on the mitochondrial enzyme aminolaevulinic acid (ALA) synthetase (Fig. 2.6) which shows increased activity. However, increased activity of ALA synthetase has now been found in all the inherited hepatic porphyrias and it has been suggested that the increase in ALA synthetase is in fact a response to increase the synthesis of intermediates to maintain normal hepatic haem levels in the face of a partial block in the synthesis of haem at different levels for each disease. Attacks are frequently precipitated by porphyrinogenic drugs (barbiturates, sulphonamides, griseofulvin, oestrogens) which cause enzyme induction in the liver, but the connection between the neurological lesions and the biochemical abnormalities is obscure.

Diagnosis is established during an acute attack by the Watson–Shwartz test for urinary porphobilinogen.

Variegate porphyria

Variegate porphyria combines the abdominal and neurological findings of acute intermittent porphyria (AIP) with chronic cutaneous photosensitivity, the latter being the dominant clinical feature of this disease which is common in South Africa. Pigmentation and hypertrichosis also occur. It is biochemically different from AIP, with continuously high faecal coproporphyrin and protoporphyrin, although during acute attacks the urinary ALA and porphobilinogen rise.

Hereditary coproporphyria

Hereditary coproporphyria is similar to the above in its sporadic acute attacks precipitated by drugs, and urinary ALA and porphobilinogen are excreted in large amounts during the attacks. The main point of distinction is the laboratory finding of raised urinary and faecal coproporphyrin levels without an equivalent increase in faecal protoporphyrin.

Porphyrinurias

The porphyrinurias are conditions in which excesses of coproporphyrin III are excreted, probably due to a block of haem synthesis between coproporphyrin III and protoporphyrin. It may be idiopathic or secondary to lead poisoning or liver disease. It is also found in some refractory anaemias.

Haem breakdown

Haemoglobin breaks down into an iron globin complex and the tetrapyrrole portion of the haem which is converted into bilirubin through a series of reactions. The bilirubin is then conjugated to bilirubin mono- and diglucuronides in the liver and excreted in the bile. In the intestine it is converted to urobilin (stercobilin) and some of it is absorbed, reduced to urobilinogen, and excreted in the urine.

If excess bilirubin is produced, as for example in haemolytic anaemia, or if it cannot be conjugated in the liver, as in premature infants and some liver disorders, then unconjugated hyperbilirubinaemia (jaundice) occurs. When jaundice results from the obstruction of bile outflow, the bilirubin in the blood is of the conjugated ('direct reacting') type.

Several uncommon forms of non-haemolytic familial jaundice have been described. Some are thought to be due to a disturbance of transport into the liver cells, some to deficiencies of the enzyme responsible for conjugation and others to disturbance of intrahepatic excretion of the conjugated pigment.

Globin metabolism

The globins of the haemoglobins are proteins made up of two identical halves which can be separated by alkali hydrolysis. Each half in turn consists of two peptide chains. In haemoglobin A these are called α and β. Each α chain contains 141 amino acids and each β chain has 146, giving a total of 574 for each molecule. Haemoglobin F (HbF) contains α and γ chains and haemoglobin A_2, α and δ chains. The synthesis and order of the amino acid sequence are under genetic control. Several allelomorphs exist for each gene controlling the four normal chains (α, β, γ and δ); each differs in its amino acid sequence. The terminal amino acids of the α chains are valyl–leucyl; of the β, valyl–histidyl–leucyl; and γ, glycyl. Delta chains are similar to α chains but have slight differences in amino acid composition. The various haemoglobin variants have differences either in the types of chain they contain or in the amino acid sequence within the chain (see

Table 2.1). The composition and properties of some of the variants will be given after consideration of the normal haemoglobins.

Haemoglobin A ($\alpha_2\beta_2$)

The whole haemoglobin A (HbA) molecule has a molecular weight of 68,000 and is elliptoid in shape. The position of the four haem units in the molecule is not known for certain. Functionally, the haem units are the sites of the reversible attachment of oxygen to the ferrous ions. This occurs in the lungs where the oxygen tension is high and each molecule of haemoglobin combines with eight atoms of oxygen to give oxyhaemoglobin (or oxygenated haemoglobin). In the tissues, where the oxygen tension is lower, some molecules give up their oxygen and become haemoglobin again. Each gramme of haemoglobin contains 3·47 mg of ferrous iron and can carry 1·34 ml of oxygen. If the blood contains 15 g/100 ml of haemoglobin then the oxygen-carrying capacity is about 20·4 ml/100 ml. The total haemoglobin content of a normal adult is about 750 g, each of the 25×10^{12} erythrocytes containing about 30 pg. The daily synthesis and release of haemoglobin is about 6·25 g. The structure of the globin moiety and the catabolism of haemoglobin have been described previously.

Haemoglobin A_2 ($\alpha_2\delta_2$)

Haemoglobin A_2 (HbA_2) is a minor component found in normal adults; it is increased in some conditions such as β-thalassaemia. The structure of this haemoglobin is not yet fully worked out; it resembles HbA and contains two δ chains instead of two β chains.

Haemoglobin F ($\alpha_2\gamma_2$)

Haemoglobin F (HbF) is found in the fetal red cells and persists in small quantities for the first few months of life. It differs from HbA in containing γ chains in place of β chains. Its physical properties differ in that it has a greater affinity for oxygen and is less positively charged in solutions at pH 8·6 and in its resistance to alkali denaturation.

Haemoglobin variants

The only differences between haemoglobins so far discovered lie in changes in the globin chain; no haem abnormality has been found to date. Disorders of globin synthesis fall broadly into two groups; in the first the synthesis of a component polypeptide chain is suppressed, whereas in the second group there is synthesized one or more abnormal polypeptide chains due to the substitution of an abnormal amino acid. The thalassaemic syndromes belong to the first group and are discussed in Chapter 3.

Most of the structurally abnormal haemoglobins are β chain variants (e.g. HbS and HbC). The pathological changes produced depend on the site of amino acid substitution and the substitution involved (see Table 2.1). Changes on the external surface of the molecule have less effect in general than those on the inside of one of the polypeptide chains or in the so-called 'haem pocket' where gross changes in stability or oxygen-carrying function are more likely to result. Sometimes these abnormal haemoglobins are classified on a functional basis into: (1) those with increased or (2) decreased oxygen affinity; (3) those such as the M haemoglobins where the affected subunit is oxidized to methaemoglobin and unable to carry oxygen; and (4) those haemoglobins which are unstable, causing a congenital non-spherocytic haemolytic anaemia.

Some of the haemoglobins can be separated from one another by electrophoresis. Because of substitution of one amino acid for another a difference of charge may be found in the molecule. If they are placed in an electric current at pH 8·6 the molecules migrate towards the positive pole. The speed with which they do this depends upon how much of a negative charge they carry. For example, HbH travels more quickly, HbF slightly more slowly, HbS moderately more slowly and HbC much more slowly than HbA (Fig. 2.7).

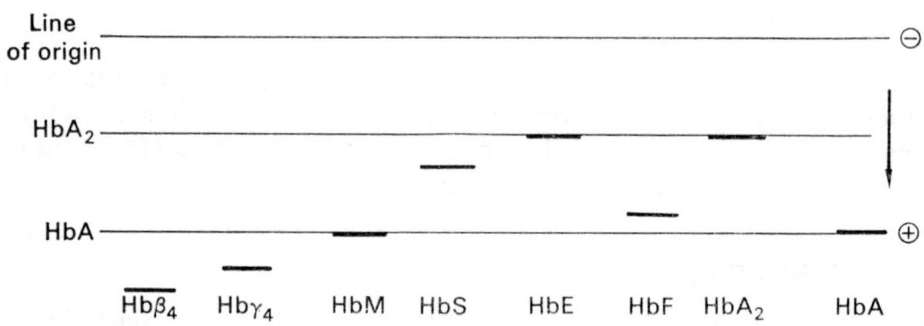

Fig. 2.7. Diagrammatic representation of haemoglobin electrophoresis.

Some haemoglobins which cannot be separated by this method may be differentiated by solubility (S and D), by electrophoresis at pH 6·5 (C and E), by movement in an ion exchange column, by lack of stability on heating or by exhibiting altered affinity for oxygen.

Haemoglobin S

Haemoglobin S is the most important of the abnormal haemoglobins because of its widespread occurrence in Negroes and the severity of the effects produced. In the reduced state this haemoglobin is poorly soluble and forms long aggregates called tactoids. If present in a red cell this may cause distortion, giving rise to sickle-shaped cells. The abnormality in this haemoglobin is due to the substitution of valine for glutamine in the sixth amino acid position from the N-terminal end. The gelling of the haemoglobin inside cells, which leads to sickling, grossly increases blood viscosity and explains the sickling 'crises' which are due to infarction in different organs (see Chapter 3).

Haemoglobin C

Haemoglobin C is similar to S, but is not associated with sickling.

Haemoglobin D

Haemoglobin D has electrophoretic properties similar to S, but differs in solubility. Recent analyses have shown that several different haemoglobins, all with the same charge but differing in amino acid sequences, are included in the term D.

Haemoglobin E

Haemoglobin E resembles C.

Haemoglobin H (β_4) *and haemoglobin Barts* (γ_4)

Haemoglobin H and haemoglobin Barts are different in that they contain tetramers of chains. Inclusion bodies of denatured protein are seen in cells containing the haemoglobin if they are stained supravitally with cresyl blue. These haemoglobins are generally found in association with α thalassaemia.

Since the letters of the alphabet have been largely used up, new haemoglobins are termed for the place of their discovery, the abnormal chain and, when known, for the chemical composition; e.g. HbS is α_2 β_2 6 val.

More details of these compounds and others found in the haemoglobinopathies are given by Huehns (1970).

Haemoglobin compounds

Haemoglobin forms a variety of compounds which may be found in the body and can be made from it in the test-tube. They can generally be recognized by their absorption spectra, an illustration of which can be found in the practical manuals.

Reduced haemoglobin

Reduced haemoglobin is normally present in the blood, accounting for about 5% of the total haemoglobin in oxygenated or 40% in reduced blood. When blood is treated with dilute ammonium sulphide or some similar mild reducing agent the oxyhaemoglobin present is reduced to haemoglobin. A reduced haemoglobin solution gives a characteristic absorption spectrum with one broad band in the green (565 nm).

Oxyhaemoglobin

Oxyhaemoglobin is normally present in the blood, accounting for 60–95% of the total haemoglobin. When fresh blood is diluted with 0·04% (w/v) of ammonia solution and shaken, the haemoglobin liberated from the cells is converted into oxyhaemoglobin by the oxygen present in the solution. This compound gives an absorption spectrum with two bands in the yellow-green (540, 578 nm). These bands may be confused with those of carboxyhaemoglobin which are, however, nearer the violet end of the spectrum.

Carboxyhaemoglobin

Although not usually present in the blood, carboxyhaemoglobin may be present following chronic or acute exposure to carbon monoxide (gas poisoning). Carbon monoxide replaces the oxygen in the molecule and thus blocks the oxygen-carrying capacity of the haemoglobin. In the test-tube it is produced by bubbling coal gas through diluted blood. The solution gives an absorption spectrum with two bands in the yellow-green (535, 572 nm). These bands may be confused with those of oxyhaemoglobin which are nearer the red end of the spectrum. The addition of a little ammonium sulphide will differentiate the two; oxyhaemoglobin is reduced to haemoglobin (one band), whereas carboxyhaemoglobin is not affected.

Methaemoglobin

When haemoglobin is oxidized, as opposed to oxygenated, the ferrous ion becomes ferric and the resulting compound is called methaemoglobin or ferrihaemoglobin. A small portion is normally present in the erythrocytes and greater quantities may be found in persons taking various drugs, such as sulphonamides. A rare condition of familial methaemoglobinaemia exists in which the erythrocytes are deficient in a factor normally required for reducing any methaemoglobin which is formed. Methaemoglobin can be reduced to haemoglobin in the body by methylene blue or ascorbic acid. In the test-tube it can be reduced to haemoglobin by ammonium sulphide. It can be produced in the test-tube by oxidation of diluted blood with a crystal of potassium ferricyanide. This solution gives an absorption spectrum with one band in the red and two in the yellow-green (630, 578, 540 nm).

Sulphaemoglobin

Sulphaemoglobin, a compound of haemoglobin the exact composition of which is not known, is found in some patients taking certain oxidative drugs. Both methaemoglobin and sulphaemoglobin may be present together in erythrocytes. Sulphaemoglobin can be produced in the test-tube by adding a small quantity of ammonium sulphide and potassium ferricyanide to diluted blood. This solution gives an absorption spectrum with a band in the red (618 nm) and continuous absorption in the yellow-green.

Sulphaemoglobin can be differentiated from methaemoglobin by the addition of ammonium sulphide. Sulphaemoglobin remains unchanged, whereas the band in the red disappears from the methaemoglobin solution due to its reduction to haemoglobin.

Haematin

Haematin is formed from haemoglobin when the globin part of the molecule is split off and the haem oxidized. Chemically it is ferrihaem. It is not usually found in the body, but may be present at the site of old haemorrhages. It is usually present in the faeces after an alimentary tract haemorrhage.

It can be produced in the test-tube by treating blood with acid or alkali. Acid solutions give an absorption spectrum with a band in the red and two fainter bands in the yellow-green (650, 582, 540 nm); alkaline solutions give a single band at the junction of red and orange (582 nm).

Haemochromogen

A colourless compound, haemochromogen is formed in the test-tube by the reduction of alkaline haematin with ammonium sulphide. It gives an absorption spectrum with two bands in the yellow-green (526, 558 nm). It is useful for identifying doubtful blood stains.

Methaemalbumin

Methaemalbumin is not normally found in the blood. Following rapid intravascular haemolysis, some of the haemoglobin present in the plasma is degraded and the haem portion becomes attached to the plasma albumin, resulting in the formation of methaemalbumin. In plasma it gives an absorption band in the red and another in the yellow-green (578, 624 nm). Because other compounds may be present, it is usual to add ammonium sulphide (Schumm's test). Any methaemalbumin present is converted into ammonium haemochromogen which has an absorption band in the yellow-green (558 nm).

Other aspects of erythrocyte biochemistry

Glucose metabolism and intracellular reductions

The erythrocyte differs from most mammalian cells in its glucose metabolism. Only glycolysis takes place, with the production of two molecules of lactate and two molecules of adenosine triphosphate (ATP) for the breakdown of one glucose molecule. The absence of respiration, which is associated with the lack of mitochondria and enzymes of the tricarboxylic acid cycle, means that not only is the released energy less efficient but also that reduced nicotinamide adenine dinucleotide phosphate (NADPH) is not available from this source. This coenzyme is necessary as a reducing agent in the prevention of oxidation of haemoglobin and other substances. It is generated in the red cells during the metabolism of glucose by an alternative pathway, the pentose–phosphate (or hexose–monophosphate) shunt, where glucose is converted to pentose through the action of two enzymes, glucose-6-phosphate dehydrogenase (G6PD) and 6-phosphogluconate dehydrogenase. For each molecule so converted one molecule of NADP is converted into the reduced form NADPH at both of the above steps (see Fig. 2.8). Lack of G6PD leads to a lowered concentration of reduced glutathione and instability of the reducing mechanisms of the cells, causing undue sensitivity to oxidizing drugs. This may lead to premature haemolysis of the erythrocytes (see p. 63).

Deficiency of G6PD was the first recognized and is the most common enzyme deficiency responsible for haemolytic anaemia in man. In the past decade other enzyme deficiencies concerned with red cell metabolism have been found to cause haemolytic anaemia. They involve deficiencies in the pathways of anaerobic glycolysis, the pentose–phosphate shunt and the reactions concerned with glutathione synthesis and reduction.

After G6PD deficiency, pyruvate kinase deficiency is the most common. This is transmitted as an autosomal recessive trait. Severity is very variable depending on zygosity but also varies due to the existence of qualitatively abnormal mutants of the enzyme, as with G6PD deficiency.

Other enzymes have been found to be deficient in rare cases and are indicated in Fig. 2.8.

The red cell membrane

The integrity of its membrane is essential for the viability of the red cell, yet the structure and function have proven difficult to elucidate due to the membrane's complexity. Its properties are dependent on its structure, which is thought to consist of a bimolecular layer of phospholipids covered on both sides by a protein layer.

The membrane is freely permeable to water and almost as permeable to univalent cations. A cation pump reverses the slow leakage of sodium ions out and potassium ions in, thus balancing the osmotic effect of intracellular haemoglobin and organic phosphates by maintaining a lowered cation concentration in the cell. The energy for the pump is provided by a

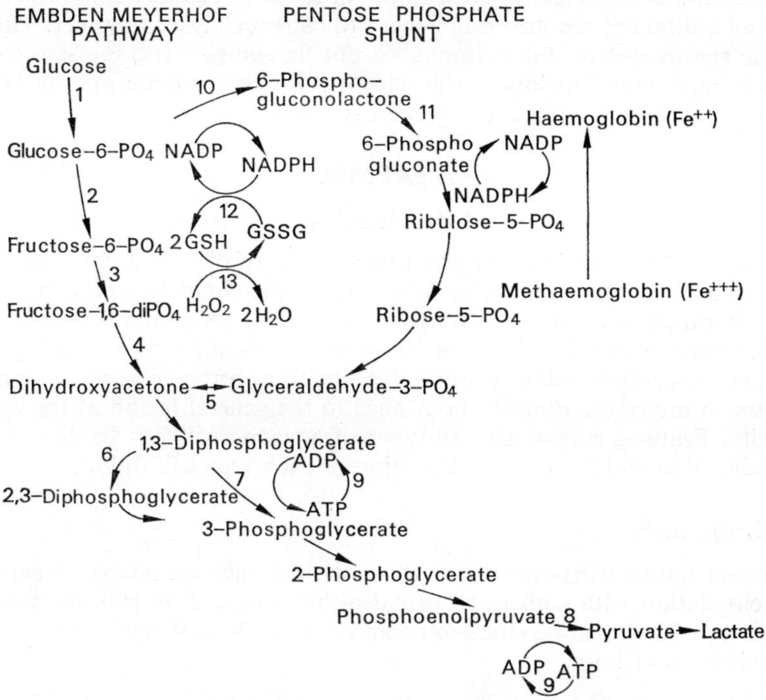

Fig. 2.8. Pathways by which glucose is metabolized in the mature red cell.

Key:

REPORTED ENZYME DEFICIENCIES

Embden-Meyerhof pathway
1. Hexokinase
2. Phosphohexose isomerase
3. Phosphofructokinase
4. Aldolase
5. Triosephosphate isomerase
6. 2,3-diphosphoglycerate mutase
7. Phosphoglycerate kinase
8. Pyruvate kinase
9. ATP-ase

Pentose Phosphate shunt
10. Glucose 6-phosphate dehydrogenase
11. 6-phosphogluconate dehydrogenase
12. Oxidized glutathione reductase
13. Glutathione peroxidase

membrane ATP-ase which requires magnesium ions and is further activated by sodium (Na^+) ions and potassium (K^+) ions. Pump failure permits ingress of sodium and water, swelling of the cell and consequent cell lysis. Some types of membrane damage, however, result in continued potassium loss without sodium gain and cell shrinkage.

Haemolysis may be of immune as well as osmotic origin. Antigens are carried on the surface of the cell membrane and when antigen–antibody reactions occur, the first component of complement is fixed to the membrane. Serum complement is a system of nine proteins which react sequentially and cause the cell to lyse by the production of defects ('holes') in the membrane with resultant disruption of the ionic equilibrium of the cell. Not all antibodies require complement to cause cell lysis, however. Those of the rhesus system, for example, do not fix complement, the sensitized cells being removed mainly by the spleen; when large amounts of antibody are present, cells are removed by the liver as well.

ANAEMIA

Introduction

Anaemia is the generic name given to a group of disorders characterized by a quantitative or qualitative deficiency of the circulating erythrocytes. The condition is common in most communities; for example, a medical practitioner in Britain might see 50 or more anaemic patients each year. Of these, four-fifths will be females. Recognition, correct classification and treatment are of the utmost importance to the general health of the community. Features common to all types of anaemia will first be described. Classification and further consideration of each type will follow.

Pathogenesis

Anaemia results whenever the erythropoietic tissues are unable to supply the circulation with sufficient normal erythrocytes. This may be due to either a deficiency in production or an excessive loss of erythrocytes or a combination of both.

Clinical features

Anaemia is characterized by pallor, palpitations, tiredness and dyspnoea. Other symptoms and signs due to anoxia or to the underlying cause of the anaemia may also be present. Anoxia may cause angina, heart failure, claudication, faintness, dizziness, headache, numbness of the extremities, renal insufficiency, pyrexia, amenorrhoea and loss of libido. Clinical features due to the underlying cause of anaemia may be found in the alimentary, nervous or reticulo-endothelial systems.

Laboratory findings

The erythrocyte count and haemoglobin concentration in the blood are usually lowered. They may be normal if there is a concomitant haemoconcentration or if the only defect is qualitative. This, however, is uncommon and the working definition of anaemia is the presence of a haemoglobin concentration below the normal level for the patient's age and sex.

Diagnosis

The diagnosis of anaemia, which may be suspected on clinical grounds, is confirmed by laboratory tests. A clinical diagnosis of a severe anaemia based on pallor is usually reliable, but this sign is not a reliable guide to moderate or mild anaemia. Estimation of the haemoglobin concentration of the blood is the most useful preliminary laboratory test. If this is below the usual values for the age and sex of the patient, then anaemia (or hydraemia) is present. Full clinical and laboratory investigations of all such patients are desirable so that the correct diagnosis and treatment can be given.

Treatment

Treatment depends upon the cause of the anaemia and this can only be determined with certainty after further tests. Generally speaking, the underlying disorder should be corrected if possible; haematinics may also be needed. If both these fail, then replacement therapy with blood transfusions is necessary.

Classification

Once anaemia has been found to be present it should be classified. Three classifications are in common use: the morphological, the aetiological and the functional (Table 2.2).

A morphological classification can be made by the examination of a well-stained blood film. Knowledge of the haemoglobin concentration, the PCV and the red cell count from which the haematological indices can be calculated may be helpful in confirming the subjective impressions made by an examination of the film. The morphological classification is of value in suggesting the likely causes of anaemia and in indicating the nature of further investigations.

An aetiological classification is of more value than a morphological classification, but is usually made only after further clinical and laboratory investigations. Unfortunately, the cause of some anaemias remains obscure and these do not readily fit into such a scheme.

A functional classification takes note of the kinetics of red cell production by the bone marrow and whether that production is effective or ineffective.

Occasionally it is convenient to group anaemias according to an age group or associated condition; for example, the anaemias of infancy and pregnancy and the anaemias due to alimentary or renal disease.

Morphological classification

In *normochromic normocytic* anaemia the erythrocyte size and staining reactions are normal but their numbers in the circulation are decreased. The MCHC, MCV and MCH are normal.

Table 2.2. Classification of anaemias

Morphological	*MCHC* (%)	*MCV* (*fl*)
1. Normochromic normocytic	32–36	76–96
2. Hypochromic normocytic	32	76–96
3. Hypochromic microcytic	< 32	< 76
4. Macrocytic	Usually normal	> 96
5. Microspherocytic	Usually normal	Normal but diameter reduced

Aetiological	
1. Increased blood loss	
(*a*) Haemorrhage	(i) Acute
	(ii) Chronic
(*b*) Haemolysis	(i) Corpuscular defects
	(ii) Extracorpuscular defects
2. Decreased blood production	
(*a*) Nutritional deficiency	(i) Iron
	(ii) Folic acid, cobalamin
	(iii) Pyridoxine
	(iv) Ascorbic acid
	(v) Protein
(*b*) Bone marrow failure	(i) Primary (idiopathic)
	(ii) Secondary to drugs, chemicals, irradiation
	(iii) Other

Functional	
1. Non-proliferative	
(*a*) Decreased marrow stimulation	(i) Endocrine disorders
	(ii) Renal disease
	(iii) Chronic infection
	(iv) Abnormal haemoglobins with decreased affinity for oxygen
(*b*) Marrow failure	(i) Marrow damage from drugs, chemicals, irradiation
	(ii) Idiopathic
(*c*) Iron deficiency	
2. Proliferative	
(*a*) Effective erythropoiesis	(i) Haemorrhage
	(ii) Haemolysis
(*b*) Ineffective erythropoiesis	(i) Folic acid, cobalamin deficiencies
	(ii) Thalassaemia, other haemoglobinopathies
	(iii) Sideroblastic
	(iv) Idiopathic refractory anaemia with hyperplastic marrow

In *hypochromic normocytic* anaemia the erythrocytes are normal in size but stain paler than usual due to a deficiency in haemoglobin. The MCHC and MCH are lowered, but the MCV is normal.

In *hypochromic microcytic* anaemia the red cells are smaller than usual as well as being pale, and all three indices are lowered.

In *macrocytic* anaemia the majority of the erythrocytes are larger than normal. The cells may stain more deeply than usual due to the increased content of haemoglobin. This is sometimes mistakenly called hyperchromia for, although the content of haemoglobin is above average, the concentration is normal. This is reflected by the value for the MCH which is raised, whereas the MCHC is normal. The MCV is increased and is usually over 100 fl. In some cases macrocytosis may be associated with hypochromia.

In *microspherocytic* anaemia the erythrocytes have a normal or only slightly reduced volume, but appear smaller because their diameter is decreased. The thickness of the cell is increased and so it appears deeply stained and without a central pale area.

Aetiological classification

The anaemias can be divided into two large groups:

1. those due to excessive loss of blood, which may be extravascular (haemorrhagic) or intravascular (haemolytic); and
2. those due to impaired production of blood due to nutritional deficiencies or failure of the bone marrow.

In some cases, both factors operate.

Functional classification

The *non-proliferative* anaemias may be due to decreased marrow stimulation, failure of the marrow itself as in aplastic anaemia, or to iron deficiency. Decreased marrow stimulation results from failure of production by the kidneys of the erythroid-stimulating hormone, erythropoietin, and is found in anaemias of renal disease, in chronic infection, endocrine disorders and in those haemoglobinopathies where the oxygen-dissociation curve is shifted to the right (decreased affinity of the haemoglobin for oxygen).

The *proliferative* anaemias are those where marrow erythroid production is increased. This may be *effective* in haemorrhagic or haemolytic anaemia or *ineffective* in anaemias where maturation defects result in the destruction of cells before their release into the circulation. This situation is encountered with the megaloblastic anaemia of cobalamin or folate deficiency, disorders of globin synthesis such as the thalassaemias and certain other haemoglobinopathies, disturbances of iron incorporation seen in the sideroblastic anaemias and in some hyperplastic anaemias of unknown cause.

Further reading

BEUTLER, E., FAIRBANKS, V. P. and FAHEY, J. L. (1963). *Clinical Disorders of Iron Metabolism.* Grune and Stratton, New York.

HUEHNS, E. R. (1970). Diseases due to abnormalities of hemoglobin structure. *Ann. Rev. Med.* **21**, 157–198.

JAFFE, E. R. (1970). Hereditary hemolytic disorders and enzymatic deficiencies of human erythrocytes. *Blood* **35**, 116–134.

KRANTZ, S. B., and JACOBSON, L. O. (1970). *Erythropoietin and the Regulation of Erythropoiesis.* University of Chicago Press, Chicago and London.

STOHLMAN, F., Jr. (1967). Some aspects of erythrokinetics. *Semin. Hemat.* **4**, 304–314.

WEATHERALL, D. J. and CLEGG, J. B. (1969). The control of human haemoglobin synthesis in health and disease. *Progr. Haemat.* **6**, 261–304.

3 Haemorrhagic and haemolytic anaemias

Introduction

The haemorrhagic and haemolytic anaemias follow excessive loss or destruction of blood when this cannot be compensated for by an increased production of red cells by the bone marrow. Although patients with moderate haemolysis or haemorrhage may maintain a normal haemoglobin concentration, anaemia usually develops if severe. Diagnosis depends on the detection of the loss or destruction of blood and on the evidence of increased erythropoiesis. Treatment is directed to the removal of the underlying cause and to replacement. The classification given in Table 2.2 forms a convenient grouping for these conditions, which are discussed here.

HAEMORRHAGIC ANAEMIAS

The haemorrhagic anaemias are due to excessive loss of blood into tissues or outside the body, which cannot be compensated by increased production of erythrocytes by the bone marrow. The possible causes of excessive bleeding are numerous and include trauma, haemoptysis, haematemesis and melaena, excessive menstruation and bleeding piles. An unusual anaemia of this type occurs in newborn babies who have 'bled' into their mothers during fetal life; even more rarely, one of a pair of twins may bleed into the other. Patients with a haemorrhagic diathesis may also develop this type of anaemia. Clinically, the haemorrhagic anaemias may be divided into acute and chronic.

Acute haemorrhage

The sudden loss of 500 ml of blood, as in blood donation, does not usually lead to any symptoms. Greater losses may be associated with shock and the loss of 1,500 ml may, depending upon the circumstances, be fatal. Following blood loss there is a constriction of the vascular bed. If the blood is examined at this time the concentration of haemoglobin and erythrocytes will be normal and the anaemia may not be apparent. However, anaemia is present since the blood volume is low. As recovery takes place, fluid is withdrawn from the tissues into the circulation and the blood volume is partially restored. Since there are no appreciable reserves of erythrocytes their concentration in the blood becomes lowered, as does the haematocrit (Fig. 3.1). If the erythrocytes were normal before the haemorrhage, then the anaemia will be normocytic and normochromic.

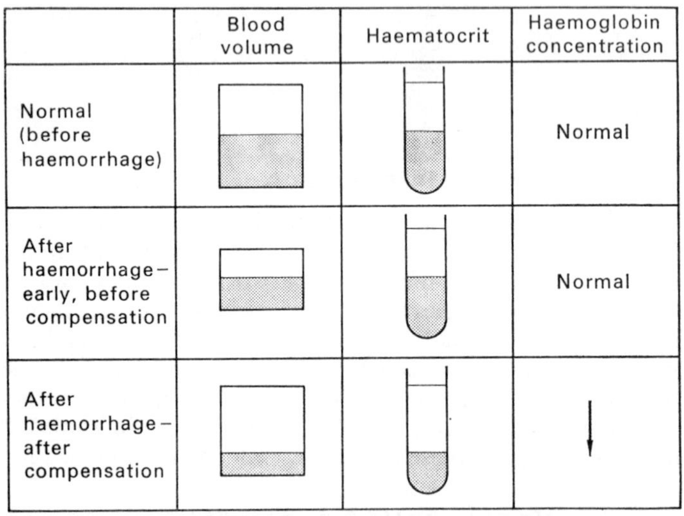

Fig. 3.1. Changes in the blood volume, haematocrit and haemoglobin in response to haemorrhage.

The resulting tissue anoxia stimulates the production of erythropoietin which in turn stimulates the bone marrow. An increased red cell production and release follows with a reticulocytosis commencing after 2 or 3 days and reaching a peak in a week or so. The proportion of new erythrocytes, usually macrocytic, in the blood rises gradually until the erythrocyte concentration and haematocrit are normal. The haemoglobin also increases but may lag behind the rise in erythrocytes with the result that there may be slight hypochromasia. The increased activity of the bone marrow is not confined to the red cells and a moderate leucocytosis and thrombocytosis may be found within a few hours of a haemorrhage. Cytological examination of the bone marrow reveals a reactive macronormoblastic hyperplasia with some increase in mitotic activity.

Treatment of shock due to blood loss is by whole blood replacement and this will help to counteract any subsequent anaemia. Plasma or plasma substitutes may be necessary whilst awaiting the cross-matching of blood. Anaemia during the recovery phase is treated by a good diet supported with iron and possibly other haematinics.

Chronic haemorrhage

In chronic blood loss the bone marrow undergoes hyperplasia and, provided it is well supplied with nutrients, anaemia does not result. The condition may be manifest, however, by a continuing reticulocytosis as well as by evidence of the actual haemorrhage. In time the continued loss leads to iron deficiency and hypochromasia becomes superimposed upon the changes due to blood loss.

An attempt should be made to find the source and correct the cause of haemorrhage. If there is no overt bleeding, a careful search for a source of occult bleeding is necessary. In women, menstrual blood loss is the commonest cause of haemorrhage leading to iron deficiency. The gastrointestinal tract is the most common source of silent bleeding in adult males and postmenopausal females. Iron treatment is given and patients may also benefit from other dietary supplements.

HAEMOLYTIC ANAEMIAS

Introduction

Normal erythrocytes have a life span of about 120 days. In haemolytic disorders this is appreciably reduced, and if the bone marrow cannot compensate, anaemia develops. Since the bone marrow has a large functional reserve, anaemia does not usually develop until the erythrocyte life span is reduced to about 20 days. In some cases bone marrow failure may be superimposed upon a haemolytic disorder, giving rise to or exaggerating the anaemia (hypoplastic crisis). Usually, however, there is evidence of both increased blood destruction and compensatory increased blood production.

Clinical features

Clinical features may be due to the anaemia, the sequelae of haemolysis and the underlying cause.

The features of anaemia have been mentioned already. Findings suggestive of haemolysis include mild jaundice, the development of biliary pigment stones, splenomegaly, a family history of anaemia or of cholelithiasis and a relationship of symptoms to drugs or chemicals. The passage of dark brown or red urine may be a sign of haemoglobinuria, suggesting intravascular haemolysis. Those features of the underlying disorder will be discussed later in the individual diseases.

Laboratory findings

Laboratory findings are produced by the increase in red cell destruction and by the compensatory rise in production of blood, together with those

Table 3.1. Differential diagnosis between haemolytic anaemias of intracorpuscular and extracorpuscular origin

	Intracorpuscular defect	*Extracorpuscular defect*
Congenital	Often	Never except in erythroblastosis fetalis
Familial	Often	Very unusual
Appearance of RBC	Characteristic malformations	No characteristic change except spherocytic and regenerative
Another disease present	Unusual	Usual
Abnormalities in Hb molecule	In the haemo-globinopathies	None found as yet
Red cell antibodies	Very rare	Frequent
Survival of transfused blood	Normal	Shortened
Survival of patient's blood in normal recipient	Shortened	Normal or better than in patient

Table 3.2. Haemolytic anaemias

Intracorpuscular defects

1. Hereditary spherocytosis
2. Haemoglobinopathies (e.g. sickle cell disease)
3. Thalassaemias
4. Sensitivity to drugs and chemicals
5. Paroxysmal nocturnal haemoglobinuria
6. Congenital non-spherocytic anaemias

Extracorpuscular defects

1. Isoimmune antibodies
   (*a*) Haemolytic disease of the newborn
   (*b*) Transfusion reaction
2. Autoimmune antibodies
   (*a*) Idiopathic (primary)
   (*b*) Symptomatic (secondary)
      (i) Lymphoproliferative disorders
      (ii) Carcinomatosis
      (iii) Connective tissue diseases (e.g. systemic lupus erythematosus)
      (iv) Drugs (e.g. methyldopa)
3. Chemicals
   (*a*) Drugs and chemicals (e.g. phenylhydrazine and lead)
4. Infections
   (*a*) Intracorpuscular parasites (e.g. malaria and bartonellosis)
   (*b*) Haemolysins (e.g. from *Cl. welchii*)
5. Physical agents
   (*a*) Burns
6. Splenomegaly
7. Microangiopathic and other fragmentary haemolytic anaemias

findings resulting from the underlying cause of the haemolysis. This lowered haemoglobin level, a raised serum unconjugated bilirubin and increased urobilinogen excretion represent increased blood destruction.

In severe cases haemoglobin, methaemoglobin and methaemalbumin may be present in the plasma and haemoglobin and its derivatives, including iron granules, in the urine. The serum haptoglobin level is usually low if there is continued haemolysis. The serum iron is usually normal or high. Red cells tagged with radioactive chromium have a decreased survival, and by scanning over the surface of the body for radioisotopic activity it may be possible to demonstrate preferential sequestration in the spleen.

The red cell morphology varies with the underlying disorder. The presence of microspherocytes, target cells or sickle cells suggests that increased haemolysis may be occurring, as also does an increased osmotic fragility of the red cells or a positive direct Coombs' test.

Evidence of increased blood production includes macrocytosis and polychromasia of the red cells. The reticulocyte count is increased and there is erythroid hyperplasia, often macronormoblastic and occasionally megaloblastic of the bone marrow if secondary folate deficiency occurs. Radioactive iron studies show rapid clearance from the plasma to the marrow with subsequent rapid incorporation into the circulating red cells due to the high rate of erythropoiesis.

Classification

The haemolytic anaemias are divided into two large groups: those in which the defect is in the red cells (intracorpuscular) and those in which the defect is extracorpuscular. Erythrocytes from a patient with an intracorpuscular defect do not survive normally in compatible healthy individuals, whilst in those with an extracorpuscular defect normal erythrocytes do not survive for the usual span of 120 days. Points which may help in differentiating these two main groups are given in Table 3.1.

The haemolytic anaemias are further classified in Tables 3.2 and 3.3.

Corpuscular defects

Hereditary spherocytosis

In hereditary spherocytosis, which is also called congenital haemolytic anaemia and familial acholuric jaundice, the defect lies in the red cells which are small and rounded. The exact biochemical lesion of the red cells is unknown but abnormalities of intracellular phosphorylation and abnormal membrane phospholipids have been described, resulting in a defect in the 'cation pump'.

Clinical features

The disorder is always inherited as an autosomal dominant character. The patients may have symptoms and signs of a mild anaemia, but often the condition is asymptomatic. A more severe anaemia may occur in 'crises' due to an exacerbation of the haemolysis or to haemolysis with superadded marrow aplasia, often associated with infections. There is a history of periodic attacks of jaundice. The spleen is generally enlarged and icterus may be detected clinically. Gall bladder pain, due to pigment stones, is not uncommon.

Table 3.3

Disease	*Genotypes*	*Haemoglobin type*
Thalassaemias		
Thalassaemia major	A A Th Th	$A + F + A_2$
Thalassaemia minor	A A Th th	$A + (F) + A_2$
Sickle cell thalassaemia	A S Th th	$S + (A) + F_2$
Haemoglobin C thalassaemia	A C Th th	C+(A)+F
Haemoglobin D thalassaemia	A D Th th	D+(A)+F
Haemoglobin E thalassaemia	A E Th th	E+(A)+F
Sickle cell anaemias		
Sickle cell anaemia	S S	S+F
Sickle cell haemoglobin C	S C	S+C+(F)
Sickle cell haemoglobin D	S D	S+D
Sickle cell haemoglobin E	S E	S+E
Haemoglobin C, D & E anaemias		
Haemoglobin C disease	C C	C+(F)
Haemoglobin D disease	D D	D+(F)
Haemoglobin E disease	E E	E+(F)
Traits		
Sickle cell trait	A S	A+S
Haemoglobin C trait	A C	A+C
Haemoglobin D trait	A D	A+D
Haemoglobin E trait	A E	A+E

Laboratory findings

The haemoglobin concentration is usually normal or slightly reduced but will be much lower during a crisis. Microspherocytes are present in the panoptically stained smears; they can be distinguished from other microcytes by the greater intensity of their staining due to the increased depth of haemoglobin in the cells. Macrocytes and polychromatic cells are also present and the reticulocyte count is usually of the order of 5–20%. The MCHC may be slightly increased. The microspherocytes have an abnormal increased osmotic fragility; they commence to lyse in a higher concentration of saline than do normal cells and haemolysis is completed at a high concentration. In the body, the microspherocytes are destroyed prematurely and survival times in the range of 14–19 days have been reported. The direct Coombs' test is negative. The osmotic fragility curve is shifted to the right (see Fig. 2.3). The serum bilirubin is usually 1–3 mg/100 ml, and the urinary and faecal urobilinogen excretion is increased.

Diagnosis

A positive family history (which is not always present), splenomegaly, the presence of microspherocytes and an increased red cell osmotic fragility allow the diagnosis to be made with comparative ease.

Treatment

Treatment is indicated if the anaemia is of sufficient severity to interfere with normal life or if there are symptoms due to biliary pigment stones. Splenectomy (and, where indicated, attention to the gall bladder) usually results in a clinical cure. No other type of treatment has been found to be of lasting benefit.

Other red cell membrane defects

A small percentage of individuals (with hereditary elliptocytosis) whose red cells are elliptical or oval in shape suffer from increased haemolysis. Other rare cases of haemolytic anaemia have been ascribed to red cell membrane enzyme or lipid deficiencies, often with several members of a family being afflicted with the disorder.

Haemoglobinopathies

The conditions which are characterized by the production of an atypical haemoglobin or by the suppression of normal haemoglobin formation are collectively called the haemoglobinopathies. Both groups are usually associated with a decreased erythrocyte survival time, hence their classification as haemolytic anaemias. They are inherited in a mendelian fashion and, whilst the presence of a single factor in the heterozygous state may cause little or no disability, the homozygous state or the double heterozygous state is usually associated with considerable morbidity.

Classification

The term haemoglobinopathy is sometimes restricted to a condition in which synthesis of an abnormal haemoglobin occurs, whereas the syndromes characterized by suppression of synthesis are called thalassaemias. Both conditions may be present simultaneously and it is probable that their underlying pathogenesis is similar. The main conditions and the haemoglobins found in them are given in Table 3.3 (see also 'Haemoglobin variants' in Chapter 2). Clinically the most important are the sickle cell anaemias and the thalassaemias.

Sickle cell anaemia (haemoglobin SS disease)

Sickle cell anaemia is a chronic haemolytic anaemia which occurs almost exclusively in Negroes. The red cells are abnormal in that they contain no HbA; it is replaced by HbS and HbF. They do not survive normally either in the host or when infused into normal recipients. The disorder is homozygous, being inherited from both parents. The heterozygous condition, sickle cell trait, is not usually associated with anaemia. However, combinations of sickle cell trait and heterozygosity for another abnormal haemoglobin may result in a condition of similar severity to sickle cell anaemia. In these conditions, however, haemoglobins other than S and F are usually present. Sickle cell anaemia is common in Negroes both in the Americas and in Africa. The presence of Negro migrants has increased the incidence of this condition in Britain. It is uncommon in Australia although the HbS trait has been found in a Caucasian family in Western Australia.

Pathogenesis

The defect in sickle cell anaemia lies in the replacement of HbA by HbS. Sickle cell haemoglobin has a valine in place of glutamic acid in the sixth amino acid residue of the β chains in the globin molecule ($\alpha^A{}_2\beta^S{}_2$ or $\alpha_2\beta^6{}_2$ val). This change results in loss of two carboxyl groups per molecule; as a result the charge of the molecule is more positive and its movement towards the positive pole on paper electrophoresis at pH 8·6 therefore is slower than that of HbA (see Fig. 2.7). Haemoglobin S forms insoluble tactoids at low oxygen tensions. The substituted valine forms a hydrophobic band with another valine, a hydrogen bond between two other amino acids being found concomitantly and, when the β chains move apart on deoxygenation, the abnormal site becomes aligned with a similar site in the chain of another molecule. As a result, cells containing it become distorted, forming crescent and sickle shapes. These erythrocytes are more susceptible to haemolysis than normal cells, but other unknown factors may also play a part in the decreased survival of the cells. The distorted cells are more viscid than normal and this may lead to thrombosis and infarction. Viscosity leads to increasing anoxia, increased sickling and increased stasis, the 'vicious viscid sickle cycle'.

Clinical features

The condition may be fatal *in utero* or in early life and the expectation of life in those who reach adulthood is much reduced. Pregnancy causes a serious maternal risk and should be avoided. The symptoms of patients with sickle cell anaemia are due to chronic anaemia, excessive haemolysis and vascular complications. Leg ulcers are often troublesome and pain due to an infarction is often a prominent symptom. The patients are usually of small stature and often have long narrow hands and feet. Bone deformities may be encountered and x-rays show a characteristic appearance due to expansion of the red marrow in the medullary space. Splenomegaly is common in infancy but the spleen usually becomes impalpable due to fibrosis following repeated infarctions. There is an increased risk of infection, mainly pulmonary, but osteomyelitis in avascular areas of infarcted bone is common and classically is due to Salmonella organisms. Poor circulation through the vasa recta of the renal medulla results in the inability to concentrate and acidify urine normally.

Laboratory findings

The anaemia is usually severe and is essentially normochromic and normocytic. A blood smear shows anisocytosis, poikilocytosis, target cells, polychromasia and often nucleated red cells. A few sickle cells may be seen but are found more easily after incubating a drop of blood with a reducing agent (usually 2% sodium metabisulphite). If a wet preparation of the reduced blood is then examined microscopically, sickle cells are readily detected. Moderate leucocytosis and thrombocytosis may be present. The bone marrow shows erythroid hyperplasia.

Haemoglobin electrophoresis shows that there is no HbA; HbS is usually predominant with a varying amount of HbF.

Diagnosis

The clinical diagnosis can be confirmed by the sickling test and paper electrophoresis of the haemoglobins present. The latter test helps to differentiate the mixed abnormalities (sickle cell–thalassaemia and sickle cell trait with other haemoglobinopathies). Family studies may also help to clarify a differential diagnosis between a homozygous and a double heterozygous state.

Treatment

There is no specific treatment. Transfusion may give temporary benefit and symptoms should be treated as they arise. Care should be taken to prevent any condition in which anoxia is likely; in particular, flying in aircraft, pressurized or otherwise, is contraindicated.

A number of methods—some quite dangerous—of preventing sickling crises have been tried with varying degrees of success claimed by their proponents. These include conversion of part of the body's haemoglobin to methaemoglobin (which does not sickle), attempts at reducing intracellular tonicity by the intravenous infusion of water, the administration of large amounts of alkali and attempted disruption of hydrophobic bands by intravenous urea infusion.

Other sickle cell disorders

Sickle cell trait

This condition, which occurs in 10–20% of Negroes, is usually asymptomatic and the total haemoglobin concentration is normal. However, about 30% of the haemoglobin present is HbS, the rest being HbA. Under conditions of anoxia, for example in unpressurized high-flying aircraft without added oxygen, sickling may occur giving rise to symptoms such as pain due to splenic infarction. Persons with sickle cell trait usually have target cells in their blood and sickle cells can be demonstrated following incubation of the blood with a reducing agent. Confirmation of the diagnosis is obtained by haemoglobin electrophoresis.

Sickle cell–haemoglobin C disease

In this condition the sickle cell trait is inherited together with that for HbC. The clinical picture is intermediate between that of sickle cell anaemia and sickle cell trait. Laboratory studies reveal sickle cells and haemoglobins C and S on electrophoresis. Sickle cell–haemoglobin D and sickle cell–haemoglobin E diseases are similar.

Sickle cell–thalassaemia

This condition resembles sickle cell anaemia clinically. Laboratory studies show more target cells in the blood smear and on electrophoresis HbA is usually present as well as HbS and HbF.

Other abnormal haemoglobin anaemias and traits

Patients homozygous for HbC and HbD and for some of the many other abnormal haemoglobins may be moderately anaemic. They show the usual features of a haemolytic disorder and target cells are often a prominent feature of the blood film. The diagnosis is made from studies of the haemoglobin by electrophoresis, solubility, chromatography and chemical analysis. Family studies are often helpful.

Individuals with abnormal haemoglobin traits (heterozygotes) are not usually anaemic unless some other abnormality is also present.

Thalassaemias

The thalassaemias are a group of disorders in which there is an inherited defect of haemoglobin synthesis. The red cells have a moderately shortened life span and for this reason the disorders are classified as haemolytic anaemias. They are characterized by a hypochromic anaemia with a normal or high level of serum and tissue iron. The MCHC is low and target cells are commonly seen. Two possible mechanisms have been suggested to explain the picture. The first is a deficient synthesis of globin and the second a deficient synthesis of haem; the latter may, however, be a secondary phenomenon. Two types of deficient globin synthesis have been recognized: in the β thalassaemias there is suppression of the synthesis of β-polypeptide chains while in the α type there is suppression of α-polypeptide chains. The condition may be homozygous or heterozygous with variable expression and may coexist with one or more of the other haemoglobinopathies. Classical thalassaemia is a β chain disorder.

Thalassaemia major (homozygous β chain type)

Thalassaemia major, a severe chronic haemolytic anaemia which is found mainly in people of Mediterranean origin, is also called Cooley's anaemia.

Pathogenesis

The red cells are abnormal in that they contain a lower concentration of HbA and, to compensate for this, increased amounts of HbF ($\alpha_2\gamma_2$) and $HbA_2(\alpha_2\delta_2)$. The erythrocytes do not survive normally in the host when infused into normal compatible recipients. The condition is homozygous, being inherited from both parents. The possibility that multiple genes may be involved is suggested by the varying pattern of the haematological disorder in the heterozygous parents. The heterozygous state usually results in a mild condition but occasionally is severe and, combined heterozygosity with that for an abnormal haemoglobin state such as HbS, gives rise to a clinical picture indistinguishable from the major disorder. The defect lies in the insufficient synthesis of the β chains and possibly in poor haem synthesis.

Clinical features

Infants with this condition fail to thrive and become progressively anaemic. They have marked hepatosplenomegaly, and expansion of the medullary cavities of the skull and facial bones gives rise to a typical 'mongoloid' appearance. Unexplained fever, leg ulcers and patchy skin pigmentation may be present. Survival into adult life is uncommon.

Laboratory findings

A moderate to severe anaemia is present. The red cells are microcytic and hypochromic in spite of normal or raised iron levels in the plasma and bone marrow. Target cells are characteristic of the condition; poikilocytosis, anisocytosis, polychromasia and basophilic stippling are usual and many nucleated red cells may be present. The erythrocytes are abnormally resistant to lysis by hypotonic saline. Electrophoresis of the haemoglobin reveals 20–90% HbF in the more severe forms, a normal or increased HA_2 and the balance of haemoglobin is HbA. The cells have a shortened survival time both in the patient and in normal recipients. The serum bilirubin is usually raised and the serum haptoglobins are reduced. The bone marrow shows hyperplasia of the erythroid tissues and an increase in the iron stores.

Diagnosis

There is no specific test which allows a diagnosis of thalassaemia to be made. A severe hypochromic anaemia with target cells occurring in the presence of a normal or high serum iron level and a high HbF level suggest the diagnosis. Family studies may be necessary to confirm the diagnosis; both parents must have thalassaemia minor.

Treatment

There is no specific treatment. Blood transfusions are required and regular transfusions inhibit increased iron absorption from the gut. Chelating agents such as desferrioxamine cannot prevent, but may slow down, the accumulation of iron in the body. Folic acid is indicated if there is a secondary folate deficiency. Other symptoms should be treated as they arise.

Thalassaemia minor (heterozygous β chain type)

Heterozygosity for the thalassaemia gene may be associated with a mild anaemia although generally symptoms are not severe. The diagnosis is suspected if there is a mild hypochromic anaemia with normal or high serum iron values. A few target cells may be seen in the film. An increased quantity of HbA_2 will be found although a subtype (normal A_2 β thalassaemia) without an increased HbA_2 content has been described. There is no definitive diagnostic test and family studies may be needed before the diagnosis can be accepted.

These patients are often given iron for years in the belief that they have a mild iron deficiency anaemia; this treatment is contraindicated unless there is an associated iron deficiency such as may occur in pregnancy. Serum iron values or examination of marrow iron reserves are helpful indicators of the need for iron therapy.

Other thalassaemias and haemoglobinopathies

An increased number of cases with a mild hypochromic anaemia not due to iron deficiency are being reported. Many of these patients are of origins other than Mediterranean but they generally fit a thalassaemia-like picture. In some cases α chain production is defective and in these individuals haemoglobins Barts ($\gamma 4$) in the newborn and H ($\beta 4$) may be found. Haemoglobin H disease is probably a doubly heterozygous condition for α thalassaemia and another, as yet unidentified, defect. Inclusion bodies of denatured HbH are found in the red cells supravitally stained with brilliant cresyl blue. Homozygous thalassaemia states probably cause death *in utero*, and the heterozygous state is not usually associated with any symptoms unless it coexists with some other haematological disorder.

Unstable haemoglobins may be associated with haemolytic anaemia and after splenectomy Heinz bodies (denatured haemoglobin) are found in the red cells. They are heterozygous states and the abnormal unstable haemoglobin forms only a small proportion of that present.

In the *Lepore haemoglobin syndrome* α chains are combined with mixed β and δ chains. *Hereditary persistence of fetal haemoglobin* is not associated with disease and is not related to the thalassaemias but may be confused with them in laboratory studies.

Other cases in which there is no evidence of defective polypeptide production are syndromes that are associated with a hypochromic anaemia not due to iron deficiency; these may be classified as thalassaemia-like states.

Enzyme deficiency haemolytic anaemias

In recent years increasing knowledge of the red cell intermediate metabolism has led to the discovery of deficiency of various enzymes associated with the clinical presence of haemolytic anaemia.

In the first-described and largest group of enzyme deficient individuals, namely those with glucose-6-phosphate dehydrogenase (G6PD) deficiency, haemolysis does not occur unless the individual is exposed to certain oxidizing drugs, fava beans or other stresses.

Glucose-6-phosphate dehydrogenase deficiency (See Fig. 2.8)

Deficiency of G6PD occurs more frequently in people of Mediterranean and Negro origin and is inherited as a sex (X)-linked character. The male hemizygote and the female homozygote more often have clinical evidence of the defect than the female heterozygote. A number of mutant variations of the enzyme have been found resulting in differing clinical features. Lack of the enzyme is more pronounced in older erythrocytes and causes lowered levels of reduced glutathione, causing a defect in the reduction mechanisms of the cell and making it more vulnerable to lysis on exposure to oxidizing drugs, chemical or plant substances. There is an increased liability to form Heinz bodies.

Lack of the enzyme is not in itself usually associated with anaemia but the ingestion of such drugs as primaquine and other antimalarial drugs, sulphones and sulphonamides results in haemolysis.

A similar state of affairs exists in favism; the ingestion of broad beans (*Vicia faba*) or inhalation of their pollen precipitates severe haemolytic anaemia within several hours, presumably due to some as yet unidentified chemical compound in the plant substance.

These agents do not cause haemolysis of enzyme-sufficient cells. Some chemicals, such as phenylhydrazine and naphthalene, may cause haemolysis even of normal cells but they act much more rapidly on enzyme-deficient cells. Since most of these substances are oxidizing agents it is thought that the cells may be damaged by oxidative drugs which cannot be reversed due to the deficient reduction in the cells.

One test for the enzyme deficiency is the incubation of the cells with phenylhydrazine; this produces large numbers of Heinz bodies. Other tests include direct enzyme assay and measurements of reduced glutathione. The tests should be carried out after the patient has recovered from the anaemia; reticulocytes and young erythrocytes usually contain adequate amounts of enzyme and these may be the only cells present after a haemolytic episode. This does not apply to favism where there is a more severe deficiency of G6PD and lowered enzyme levels are found even in reticulocytes.

Pyruvate kinase deficiency

Pyruvate kinase deficiency, which is inherited as an autosomal recessive character, may be associated with haemolytic anaemia. It is second in frequency to G6PD deficiency and was the first enzyme deficiency described associated with the Embden–Meyerhof glycolytic pathway (G6PD deficiency involves the hexose–monophosphate shunt). Considerable heterogeneity in both its clinical severity and the biochemical abnormality are known to occur. In general, homozygotes suffer from fairly severe disease with a haemoglobin in the range of 6–12 g/100 ml and moderate to marked reticulocytosis. Spherocytes are absent and the osmotic fragility test is normal. Small numbers of acanthocytes are frequently found.

Erythrocytes of homozygotes show 5–25% of normal activity on pyruvate kinase assay, but this does not correlate well with the degree of haemolysis found clinically. Enzyme assays have shown that a 'pile-up' of intermediates occurs proximal to the defective point of glycolysis. As with G6PD deficiency, pyruvate kinase deficiency includes cases where qualitative aberrations of the enzyme occur.

Splenomegaly is usual in pyruvate kinase deficiency, and in selected cases splenectomy may result in amelioration of transfusion requirements.

Other enzyme deficient anaemias

In addition to G6PD deficiency which may be considered a prototype of enzyme deficiency affecting the pentose-phosphate shunt and pyruvate kinase deficiency, the first-described abnormality of the Embden–Meyerhof pathway, a number of other enzyme deficiencies have now been described, sometimes only in individual patients, affecting both of these pathways and also involving enzymes directly concerned with the integrity of the glutathione reduction system. These are indicated in Fig. 2.8.

The clinical picture produced in these conditions is similar to that of homozygous pyruvate kinase deficiency.

Paroxysmal nocturnal haemoglobinuria

A rare disorder, paroxysmal nocturnal haemoglobinuria is characterized by intravascular haemolysis, leucopenia and thrombocytopenia. The haemolysis and haemoglobinuria usually occur more markedly following sleep. The patient's erythrocytes have a shortened survival time in normal recipients; furthermore, they are haemolysed by normal serum if it is acidified to pH 6·5 (Ham's test). However, in some cases, stimuli other than sleep (such as iron therapy) appear to initiate a haemolytic episode. In addition to the normal features of a haemolytic anaemia, haemoglobinaemia, methaemoglobinaemia, haemoglobinuria and haemosiderinuria will be present. The Coombs' antiglobulin test is negative.

The nature of the red cell defect is not known for certain. The red cells are abnormally sensitive to the lytic action of complement, presumably due to a membrane defect. A deficiency of membrane acetylcholinesterase has been described but it is not specific for the disease.

Extracorpuscular defects

Isoimmune haemolytic disorders

In isoimmune haemolytic disorders the red cells are coated with antibodies developed in the body of another human being. Since this is an antibody within the same species, it is called an isoantibody.

Haemolytic disease of the newborn

Haemolytic disease of the newborn is due to premature destruction of fetal red cells by isoantibodies formed in the mother and which subsequently cross the placental barrier. The effect varies from a mild anaemia to a severe condition in which the fetus is killed. Severe forms are usually associated with repeated sensitization by the Rh-positive (D) antigen. Milder forms are seen following A and B incompatibilities. Other blood group antigens are occasionally involved.

Rh D incompatibility

About 10% of Rh-negative women who carry Rh-positive babies (the D antigen having been inherited from the father) develop antibodies. The fetal red cells which enter the maternal circulation during pregnancy or at delivery stimulate the production of antibodies. These antibodies may subsequently cross the placental barrier and enter the fetal circulation. Here they coat the erythrocytes which are subsequently prematurely destroyed. Unless the mother has previously been sensitized by a blood transfusion or previous pregnancy, the condition generally is mild. In successive pregnancies, however, the chances of the fetus being affected are greater, rising from 1 in 150 for the first pregnancy to 1 in 15 for the second and about 1 in 10 for subsequent pregnancies. If the father is heterozygous for the Rh factor (genotype Dd) the chances are that half the children will be Rh-negative and not affected. In severe cases the anaemia may cause the death of the fetus, resulting in a stillbirth. If the serum bilirubin is very high, damage to the basal ganglia of the brain (kernicterus) may occur and children so affected frequently die within a week of birth. The jaundice is usually more marked in premature infants and is partially due to the immaturity of the liver which cannot readily conjugate the bilirubin to its non-toxic glucuronide. Kernicterus can be prevented by exchange transfusion in which the baby's blood is replaced by donated Rh-negative blood.

In addition to the usual feature of a haemolytic anaemia the blood contains numerous nucleated red cells. The direct Coombs' antiglobulin test is positive; that is, the erythrocytes washed three times in saline to remove any plasma are agglutinated by an anti-human globulin serum because the red cells are coated with antibody γ-globulin.

The maternal serum also contains antibodies. Sometimes these cause agglutination of Rh-positive cells suspended in saline, in which case the antibody is called a 'complete' or saline-agglutinating antibody. Often they can only be demonstrated by suspending the Rh-positive cells in albumin or by testing the serum by incubating it with donor erythrocytes containing known antigens and then testing this with an anti-human globulin serum (indirect Coombs' test). In this case the antibodies are called 'incomplete'.

ABO incompatibility

This occurs when babies of groups A, B or AB are carried by group O mothers. Anti-A or anti-B crossing the placental barrier may affect the red cells but any anaemia which results is not usually severe. The incidence of the disease depends upon the criteria used for diagnosis, and figures varying from 1 in 100 to 1 in 1,000 pregnancies have been reported. The more severe cases are usually due to anti-A. The Coombs' test is usually negative or only weakly positive. The washed cord blood cells sediment rapidly when suspended in the polyvinyl pyrrolidine mixture. This feature has been suggested as a means of diagnosis and a measure of the severity of the condition.

Prevention of haemolytic disease of the newborn

Any event which increases the number of fetal cells entering the circulation of a susceptible mother can potentiate the severity of rhesus isoimmunization and hence amniocentesis, external version, manual removal of the placenta and caesarian section should be carried out only when absolutely indicated. The most important way of preventing rhesus isoimmunization is the administration of anti-D immunoglobulin upon delivery or after any incident or procedure liable to result in isoimmunization. The risk of isoimmunization can be reduced by 90% by giving anti-D antiserum to all Rh-negative women who have an Rh-positive child.

Treatment of haemolytic disease of the newborn

Management of the patient sensitized with anti-Rh antibody during pregnancy involves monitoring of the titre of the antibody, in certain cases aspiration of amniotic fluid for spectrophotometric analysis of products of haemoglobin breakdown and early induction of labour. In severely affected cases where fetal death will occur before premature induction of labour is possible, intrauterine transfusion of the fetus may be performed.

In the affected infant severe hyperbilirubinaemia or anaemia is treated by exchange transfusion in which group O Rh-negative cells are given. Other methods for treating less severe grades of jaundice, such as exposure to ultraviolet light and hepatic enzyme induction by the use of phenobarbitone, have been tried.

Incompatible blood transfusions

Haemolysis of donor blood may occur if the recipient's plasma contains an antibody to an antigen in the transfused red cells. Less commonly, antibodies (usually high titre anti-A haemolysins) in the donor blood may cause haemolysis of the recipient's cells. The occurrence of haemolysis due to these causes should be avoided by carrying out appropriate compatibility tests before all blood transfusions.

Autoimmune haemolytic disorders

In autoimmune haemolytic disorders the patient's erythrocytes are prematurely destroyed because they are coated with autoantibodies. Anaemia may result and can be classified clinically into acute or chronic and according to whether the condition is primary (idiopathic) or secondary (symptomatic) to some other disease. It may also be classified according to the nature of the antibodies present.

The anaemia occurs if the bone marrow is unable to compensate for the increased destruction of the red cells and is severe and acute if haemolysis is massive. In some cases anaemia develops or is accentuated by an associated bone marrow hypoplasia or megaloblastosis due to secondary folate deficiency.

The mechanisms of red cell destruction vary with the type of antibody. If the antibodies are most active at 37°C (warm type) the red cell agglutinates are trapped in the spleen and other reticular tissues where they are lysed and phagocytosed. Warm type antibodies are usually IgG and do not fix complement in order to cause cell lysis. If the antibodies are most active at lower temperatures (cold type) there may be intravascular haemolysis or agglutination more especially in the peripheral tissues. These antibodies belong to the IgM class and always fix complement, although sera vary in their ability to cause lysis.

Clinical features

The clinical findings are those of a haemolytic anaemia and possibly also those of an underlying disorder. The anaemia may be very rapid in onset with severe constitutional disturbance or may develop insidiously over many months. Jaundice and splenomegaly are common. Acute episodes of haemolysis may be accompanied by haemoglobinaemia and haemoglobinuria. Where cold antibodies are present, autoagglutination of cells in peripheral blood vessels causes the cold haemagglutinin syndrome of peripheral cyanosis, vascular complications suggesting Raynaud's phenomenon, peripheral thrombosis and gangrene. If the cold antibody has a wide thermal amplitude, continuous haemolysis is often present.

Laboratory findings

As well as the findings common to all the haemolytic anaemias, there may be spherocytosis and an increased erythrocyte osmotic fragility. Antibodies on the cells are demonstrated by the direct Coombs' test which is positive. Antibodies may also be demonstrated in the serum (indirect Coombs' test). Both these and antibodies eluted from the red cell surfaces may be tested for thermal range, globulin type and antigen specificity. By testing at 37°C and 20°C they can be divided into warm and cold types. The globulin type of the antibody is tested for, seeing if the cells are agglutinated by anti-human globulin antibody from which the anti-γ-globulins have been absorbed. If they are the antibodies of the non-γ type they are usually most active in the 'cold'.

The antibody specificity is tested by examining its ability to coat erythrocytes of different antigen phenotypes. In the majority of cases of warm antibody haemolytic anaemia, specificity against Rh antigens is found. Recently it has been discovered that many of the so-called non-specific IgM cold antibodies are specific for the I antigen present in the erythrocytes of most people. In some cases associated with a cold antibody the Wassermann reaction may be falsely positive. In the rare disease, paroxysmal cold haemoglobinuria, the cold antibodies absorbed on to red cells at low temperatures cause haemolysis when warmed. This is seen *in vitro* in the Donath–Landsteiner reaction. In this disease the cold antibody is IgG and has anti-P specificity.

Idiopathic autoimmune haemolytic anaemia

Only if all the known causes of acquired autoimmune haemolytic anaemia have been excluded can the idiopathic type be diagnosed. It is therefore a retrospective diagnosis. The reason for the formation of antibodies in such cases is not known; it may be due to a breakdown of immunological tolerance or to a fault in the red cell surface which alters it to such an extent that it becomes antigenic. Most cases are associated with antibodies of the warm type. The condition may be acute or chronic. Acute cases are common in childhood (Lederer's anaemia) and after a severe illness the disease often becomes quiescent. Although some deaths occur the prognosis is generally good. In adult cases both acute and chronic types are found. The acute types are severe and have an appreciable mortality. They may become chronic or a remission may occur.

Treatment

Steroid therapy is usually advised as the first line of treatment, but should not be given for more than a few months unless there is no other way of controlling the condition. A starting dose of 50–75 mg of prednisone should be used and the dosage reduced after a week or two depending upon the response of the patient. Splenectomy is often of benefit and is still advised by some as the first line of treatment. Some guide as to the benefit of splenectomy may be gained by measuring the uptake of radioactive labelled erythrocytes in the spleen and liver. A high uptake in the spleen suggests that splenectomy might be helpful. However, it may be beneficial even if sequestration of erythrocytes cannot be demonstrated. It is indicated whenever control by steroids is difficult or prolonged.

The third line of treatment is the use of immunosuppressive agents in order to depress antibody production by antibody-producing cells. Azathioprine has been most often used in warm type autoimmune haemolytic anaemia where the use of steroids and splenectomy occasionally fail to induce a remission. In cold antibody haemolytic anaemia the response to steroids and splenectomy is usually poor and chlorambucil has been found to achieve remission in some of these cases.

Secondary autoimmune haemolytic anaemia

An autoimmune haemolytic anaemia may be found in association with a large variety of other conditions; the commoner ones are mentioned below.

The leukaemias and lymphomas may be complicated by haemolytic anaemia. In particular, patients with chronic lymphocytic leukaemia frequently show evidence of haemolysis. It is possible that the neoplastic lymphoreticular cells produce an abnormal antibody against the red cells. The management of such a patient is that of treating the underlying disorder and haemolysis may be controlled with corticosteroids; occasionally, splenectomy may be required.

Disseminated lupus erythematosus is not infrequently associated with a warm-type autoimmune haemolytic anaemia. A search for lupus erythematosus cells should be made in all cases of autoimmune haemolytic anaemia. Treatment is with corticosteroids, which may control both the underlying disorder and the anaemia.

Infections such as Mycoplasma pneumonia and infectious mononucleosis may be associated with an autoimmune haemolytic anaemia during the acute stage of the disease or a few weeks later. A cold agglutinin is often detectable in such cases. It is thought that the antibody is formed against red cells which have been altered in some way by the virus. If haemolysis is severe, steroids may control it until a spontaneous remission occurs. Occasionally, splenectomy is necessary.

Miscellaneous conditions associated with this type of anaemia include various carcinomas, tuberculosis, regional ileitis, sarcoidosis and periarteritis nodosa. Certain drugs can cause an autoimmune haemolytic anaemia (see below).

Chemicals and drugs

Phenylhydrazine, naphthalene and the sulphones may be associated with a haemolytic anaemia even if the erythrocytes are metabolically normal. Many of these agents appear to act by causing oxidative changes in the cells which cannot be reversed; as a consequence, where there is a deficiency of the reduction mechanisms (e.g. in G6PD deficiency) cells are more sensitive to these agents. The blood picture is that of a haemolytic disorder; spherocytosis, basophilic stippling and fragmentation may be seen. Heinz bodies are commonly present in the erythrocytes. Methaemoglobin and sulphaemoglobin may be present in the blood.

There are three *immune* haemolytic reactions which may be produced by drugs.

1. *The 'innocent bystander' reaction* is one in which an antibody can be produced against a number of agents such as the sulphonamides, quinine and quinidine, and combines with the antigen in the circulation. The resultant complex binds to the red cells by passive absorption and leads to complement activation and cell lysis.

2. *The penicillin type of reaction* is seen following high doses of penicillin or one of the cephalosporins and is due to binding of the drug and an antibody (IgG) formed against the drug to the red cell membrane. This results in a positive Coombs' test of the IgG type and haemolysis in some patients.

3. *The reaction produced to α-methyldopa* is due to the production of an IgG antibody, usually with Rh specificity, which is indistinguishable from the antibody found in the warm type of idiopathic autoimmune haemolytic anaemia. The incidence of a positive direct Coombs' test in patients receiving α-methyldopa depends on the dose and length of exposure but is of the order of 10–20% after 6 months. Actual haemolysis occurs in only 0·1% or so of these with positive Coombs' tests.

Lead intoxication is frequently complicated by an anaemia. This is due to enzymatic blocks in haem synthesis by inhibition of ALA synthetase, ALA dehydratase and haem synthetase (see Fig. 2.6), as well as an accelerated destruction of erythrocytes in the circulation. Basophilic stippling of the erythrocytes is a special feature of lead poisoning and persons exposed to lead in their work should undergo regular blood tests. Those with coarsely stippled erythrocytes should be further investigated. Bone marrow examination in lead poisoning often reveals ringed sideroblasts.

Urinary coproporphyrin and ALA excretion are increased and correlate well with the clinical assessment, while the blood lead level is less reliable and urinary lead excretion shows a poor correlation. The erythrocytes will show a markedly elevated protoporphyrin content and a slightly elevated coproporphyrin content.

Physical agents

Burns may be associated with an intravascular haemolysis severe enough to cause anaemia. Cold may precipitate haemolytic crises in patients whose plasma contains cold autoimmune antibodies.

Infections

In malaria and bartonellosis the erythrocytes are invaded by the micro-organism and thus destroyed. If these infections are severe, haemolytic anaemia will result. In *Clostridium welchii* infections the organisms may produce sufficient haemolysins to cause an acute haemolytic anaemia. Haemolysis may also be found in severe staphylococcal infection.

Hypersplenism

Enlargement of the spleen, for whatever reason, may be associated with a pathological increase in its normal function of removing erythrocytes from the circulation. As a result, the life cycle of the cell is reduced and, if this is severe, may cause an anaemia. In such cases there is frequently a concomitant neutropenia and thrombocytopenia. Depression of the bone marrow may be present at the same time due to a humoral factor secreted by the spleen.

Microangiopathic and other fragmentary haemolytic anaemias

The terms microangiopathic and fragmentary have been applied to those haemolytic anaemias which occur in conditions such as disseminated malignant disease and uraemia when haemolytic antibodies cannot be demonstrated. Cell survival studies reveal a shortened life span but decreased production may also play a part in the production of the anaemia. Diseased vascular endothelium with or without local fibrin deposition damaging red cells during contact is thought to be significant in the pathogenesis of the microangiopathic haemolytic anaemia in which fragmented and irregularly shaped red cells are seen. Some cases are accompanied by thrombocytopenia and other evidence of intravascular coagulation. Thrombotic thrombocytopenia, renal cortical necrosis, glomerulonephritis, metastatic malignancy (especially mucin-forming adenocarcinoma), malignant hypertension, severe pre-eclampsia and eclampsia are the usual underlying disorders. A similar picture may be found if blood comes in contact with the rough surface of an intravascular prosthesis. In some instances thrombocytopenia is present and this is common in an ill-defined condition, called the haemolytic uraemic syndrome, occurring in infants.

The aetiology of the underlying vascular disease may be obvious, as in malignant hypertension, or obscure, as in the haemolytic uraemic syndrome. Nevertheless, the recognition of the importance of intravascular coagulation as the cause of the microangiopathy in some patients has led to the use of heparin therapy with some success. When irreversible renal damage has occurred, little success can be hoped for. If intravascular coagulation is secondary to an underlying vascular disease, heparin may be of temporary benefit if the primary disease can be controlled.

Further reading

BRAIN, M. C. (1971). The red cell and haemolytic anaemia. In: *Recent Advances in Haematology*, 146–194. Ed. by A. Goldberg and M. C. Brain. Churchill Livingstone, Edinburgh and London.

DACIE, J. V. and WORLLEDGE, SHEILA M. (1969). Autoimmune hemolytic anemias. *Progr. Hemat.* **6**, 82–120.

VALENTINE, W. H. (1970). The hereditary hemolytic anemias associated with erythrocyte enzyme deficiencies. *Advanc. intern. Med.* **16**, 303.

4 Iron deficiency anaemia

Introduction

The first recorded use of iron in Medicine is found in ancient Hindu medical practice. The Greek physicians equated iron with strength and treated weakness in patients with water in which old swords had been left to rust. In the seventeenth century, Thomas Sydenham used iron and steel filings steeped in Rhenish wine for the treatment of chlorosis, an old name for iron deficiency anaemia.

Iron deficiency anaemia is the commonest form of anaemia in the world today, not only in the developing countries but also in Western society.

Iron for haemoglobin synthesis is available from the absorption of dietary iron and from the iron reserves of the body. If the requirements or losses of iron are greater than the amount absorbed from the diet then the reserves become depleted. Decreased levels of iron-containing enzymes and degenerative changes in epithelial tissue may follow, and if the deficiency persists anaemia will develop.

Iron deficiency anaemia is therefore found when there is inadequate intake of food iron, poor absorption or excessive demands or losses. Frequently, more than one factor plays a part. Nevertheless, the most common factor causing iron deficiency in Western countries is blood loss.

Failure of incorporation of iron into haemoglobin in thalassaemia and some other hypochromic anaemias gives a false picture of iron deficiency; since stainable iron is present in the marrow and the serum iron is not decreased, such conditions should not be classified as iron deficient.

Normal iron balance

In the absence of blood loss, the iron content of the body generally remains stable throughout adult life. The sources, absorption and metabolic fate of iron are discussed in Chapter 2.

Recent studies have shown that foods with a given iron content vary in the amount of their iron available for absorption. Iron from food of animal origin is usually better absorbed than that in cereals, but individual exceptions occur; for example, the iron in egg yolk is poorly absorbed. Food iron is less readily absorbed than iron in organic salts. Another factor is the interaction which occurs between foods. The absorption of iron from an individual eating an egg may be increased two to three times by 100 ml of orange juice (which only contains 50 mg ascorbic acid). Fructose is also known to increase iron absorption; food phosphates, oxalates and phytates, however, decrease iron availability by the formation of insoluble iron salts. Iron cooking-pots may contribute significantly to the iron intake, as may various beverages, notably red wine.

It has been calculated that a refined Western diet contains 6 mg iron for each 1,000 calories, thus yielding 15 mg each day to a normal adult male, of which only 0·5–1·0 mg will actually be absorbed. The basal loss of iron in the adult male is 0·5–1·0 mg, thus maintaining a balance. The average menstrual loss in a female adds a further 0·5 mg per day, and is often greater. To this must be added the additional average total iron requirement of pregnancy, which is around 700 mg. Although lactation results in a further 0·5–1·0 mg loss of iron each day, this is usually nullified by amenorrhoea during lactation.

The rapid growth of infancy and early childhood increases the daily iron requirement by approximately 1·0 mg and a similar need develops when adolescence results in a period of rapid growth. The status of iron stores of an individual also regulates absorption, which is increased in iron deficiency.

Pathogenesis of iron deficiency

Women go through life, especially in their reproductive years, with a precarious iron balance and generally have diminished iron reserves compared to men, making them more vulnerable to any lack of dietary iron or excessive losses.

Lack of dietary iron

Milk is a poor source of iron, and deficiency may develop in babies fed for a prolonged period on milk alone. Normal full-term babies contain a reserve of iron which is used up by about 3 months if supplements are not given. Twins and prematurely born infants have decreased iron reserves.

In adults, a poor diet alone is an uncommon cause of iron deficiency but often contributes to anaemia mainly due to some other factor. The diet of old persons living alone, of food faddists and of some therapeutic regimens may lack iron.

Poor absorption

Disorders of the gut may result in defective iron absorption. Partial or total gastrectomy is a common cause of iron deficiency due to bleeding, atrophic gastritis, mechanical bypass of the duodenum, a rapid transit time and dietary faddism from post-gastrectomy symptoms. Atrophic gastritis with achlorhydria is frequently associated with iron deficiency. Antacids such as calcium carbonate, aluminium hydroxide and magnesium hydroxide interfere with iron absorption. Disease of the upper intestine may also cause poor absorption. Pica such as the eating of clay (geophagia) or of starch has been shown to impair iron absorption. It is not always clear whether the iron deficiency is the cause or the result of this habit.

Extra physiological needs

The rapid growth of infancy and adolescence may give rise to iron deficiency and anaemia is not uncommon in both sexes; the onset of menstruation in females is an additional factor. During pregnancy, prophylactic iron therapy is required because of the additional requirements.

Haemorrhage

The commonest cause of iron deficiency is loss of iron from haemorrhage. In women, menorrhagia is the most important cause. In males and post-menopausal females, bleeding into the intestinal tract is commonest. Peptic ulceration and haemorrhoids are frequent causes; carcinoma of the stomach or colon may present with an iron deficiency anaemia without localizing symptoms or signs. Hookworm and other parasitic infestations are important causes of blood loss in tropical countries.

Sequestration of iron

In certain rare diseases, iron may accumulate in certain organs and not be available for haemoglobin synthesis. In pulmonary haemosiderosis iron accumulates in the lung, causing iron deficiency anaemia, and a similar situation can occur in Goodpasture's syndrome. One case has been described of a child with complete absence of the iron transport protein, transferrin, which resulted in iron deficiency anaemia but excessive organ deposition of iron.

Clinical features

The symptoms and signs of iron deficiency anaemia may be due to iron deficiency, to anaemia or to an underlying disorder. Mild anaemia may be present without any definite symptoms. Usually there is an insidious onset. In infancy and childhood, pallor and general debility with increased liability to infections are common, In adults, a frequent complaint is lack of energy and in many cases pallor will be obvious. Anoxia may precipitate such symptoms as cardiac angina or congestive heart failure and claudication. In a small proportion of cases the spleen may be slightly enlarged and changes due to iron deficiency in the epithelial tissue may be present. These include thin and brittle nails, a smooth tongue and angular stomatitis ('perlèche'). In women with chronic iron deficiency there may be dysphagia due to the formation of a mucosal web at the upper end of the oesophagus (Plummer–Vinson or Paterson–Kelly syndromes). In South Wales, where this syndrome is very common, recent epidemiological studies have suggested that the occurrence of the oesophageal web and iron deficiency may be fortuitous. Disturbances of menstruation are common and pruritus vulvae is an occasional symptom. Symptoms and signs due to an underlying disorder, such as a peptic ulcer or haemorrhoids, may be present.

Laboratory findings

Blood

In early and mild cases of iron deficiency anaemia the erythrocytes may be comparatively normal both in size (normocytosis) and numbers, but they are hypochromic. The average haemoglobin concentration (MCHC) and content (MCH) of each erythrocyte is lowered, the MCHC being less than 32% and the MCH less than 27 pg.

In later and more severe cases the erythrocytes are also smaller than usual (microcytic), having a reduced MCV (below 76 fl). Stained smears show poikilocytosis and anisocytosis as well as the hypochromasia and microcytosis. The haemoglobin concentration is below normal but rarely less than 6 g/100 ml of blood, the erythrocyte count between 3 and 5 million/μl and the PCV 25–40%. The erythrocytes may show slightly increased resistance to lysis by hypotonic saline. The reticulocyte count is usually normal or slightly increased; larger numbers of young cells (reticulocytes) may be present if haemorrhage is occurring. The serum iron content is lower than normal and the serum iron-binding capacity increased (Fig. 2.5).

Bone marrow

The bone marrow shows erythroid hyperplasia if the cause of iron deficiency is haemorrhage; the normoblasts are smaller than normal with irregularly shaped and poorly stained cytoplasm. The marrow iron stores are absent.

Diagnosis

Iron deficiency anaemia is often diagnosed in general practice on clinical grounds, an iron preparation given and a therapeutic response accepted as confirming the diagnosis. However, laboratory confirmation of the clinical diagnosis is preferable and a haemoglobin estimation and blood film examination should be carried out. If there is any doubt as to the diagnosis or if response to treatment is inadequate the PCV should be determined and the MCHC worked out; levels below 30% suggest iron deficiency. Further tests which may be needed include serum iron and iron-binding capacity (transferrin) estimations and bone marrow examination for cytology and the assessment of stainable iron stores. These will help to differentiate simple iron deficiency from the thalassaemias and sideroblastic anaemias in which hypochromasia is combined with normal or high serum iron and adequate iron stores in the bone marrow. An iron absorption test may be helpful if malabsorption is suspected.

Treatment

The underlying cause of the anaemia should be corrected as soon as possible and an iron preparation given. Oral iron is usually best but parenteral preparations can be given if there are special indications (see below).

Oral preparations

Tablet (see Table 4.1)

The preparation of choice is ferrous sulphate. Each 200 mg tablet of the dried salt and each 300 mg tablet of the hydrated salt provides approximately 60 mg of elemental iron. For most patients with iron deficiency anaemia a practical daily dosage of elemental iron is 100–200 mg, which

Table 4.1. Iron preparations for oral use

Tablets		*Elemental iron content*	*Usual adult dose*
Ferrous sulphate (hydrated)	300 mg	60 mg	1 t.d.s. between meals
Ferrous sulphate (dried)	200 mg	60 mg	1 t.d.s. between meals
Ferrous gluconate	300 mg	40 mg	1 t.d.s. between meals
Ferrous fumarate	200 mg	60 mg	1 t.d.s. between meals
Ferrous succinate	150 mg	35 mg	2 t.d.s. between meals
Liquids		*Elemental iron content*	*Usual adult dose*
Ferric ammonium citrate		18 mg/ml	Adults: 200 mg iron daily Children: 2 mg/kg daily (all liquids)
Ferrous sulphate syrup		8 mg/ml	
Ferrous sulphate drops		25 mg/ml	
Ferrous gluconate elixir		6 mg/ml	
Ferrous succinate		30 mg/ml	

is provided by one tablet three times daily (t.d.s.). Absorption of iron is increased if the tablets are taken on an empty stomach without food and if they are taken more than 4 hours apart.

Patients frequently complain of side-effects due to iron, often because of traditional attitudes towards iron therapy. Reactions to iron include nausea, vomiting, cramps, diarrhoea, constipation and, occasionally, sweating and syncope. Side-effects are almost invariably dose-related and not due to the preparation used. Reduction of the dose or taking the tablet with food will often abolish them. To circumvent the side-effects, a large number of different iron preparations have been introduced, which are more expensive; these include ferrous gluconate, ferrous fumarate and ferrous succinate. These tablets usually contain lower doses of elemental iron. Adjuvants such as ascorbic acid, succinate, hydrochloric acid, cobalt or emulsifying agents may effect some increase in absorption but add considerably to the cost. The introduction of enteric-coated and slow release preparations of ferrous sulphate carry the iron past the duodenum and upper jejunum where most iron is normally absorbed, thus decreasing side-effects by decreasing absorption.

Iron poisoning may occur in children if they swallow a large number of iron tablets (which are frequently sugar-coated and attractive in colour) and patients should be warned to keep them in a safe place. The recent introduction of push-through foil packaging, although expensive, makes the ingestion of a large number of tablets difficult for an infant.

Liquid

Some patients who will not take tablets can take iron in the form of fluid. Suitable preparations include ferric ammonium citrate, ferrous sulphate and ferrous gluconate (Table 4.1).

Patients should be treated from 2 months to 1 year following a return of the haemoglobin to normal levels so as to replace their iron reserves. Those women who have a tendency to become iron deficient should be advised to take iron for 1 week every month.

Parenteral (see Table 4.2)

Failure to respond to oral iron therapy usually indicates that the patient is not taking the tablets or that the diagnosis of iron deficiency was wrong. Sometimes the amount of iron prescribed is insufficient to replace the amount being lost. Parenteral iron is indicated in certain diseases of the gut such as malabsorption or ulcerative colitis where the iron may aggravate the colitis, or where the patient's requirement of iron exceeds that which can be given by mouth and in the last 3 months of pregnancy.

Intramuscular iron preparations have been used for a number of years. The preparation of choice is iron dextran (Imferon). An alternative preparation is an iron–sorbitol–citric-acid complex stabilized with dextrin (Jectofer). Both these preparations contain 50 mg of iron per ml. Two millilitres of either is given by deep intramuscular injection into the upper outer quadrant of the buttocks, using a 'Z-track technique' to avoid subcutaneous staining with iron, every day or every other day to a total dosage calculated from the following formula:

200 mg for each g/100 ml of haemoglobin deficiency

plus

1,000 mg to replace the body stores,

or

$$0{\cdot}6 \times \text{body weight in kg} \times \left(\frac{100\text{-Hb in g/100 ml}}{14{\cdot}8}\right) \text{mg}$$

Table 4.2. Parenteral iron preparations

		Elemental iron/ml	*Route*
Dextran iron (Imferon)	Ferric hydroxide + dextran (mol. wt. 180,000)	50 mg	I.M. or I.V.
Dextrin iron (dextriferron) (Astrafer)	Ferric hydroxide + dextrin (mol. wt. 230,000)	20 mg	I.V.
Iron sorbitol citrate (Jectofer)		50 mg	I.M.

Intravenous treatment predated intramuscular therapy but the saccharated iron oxide which was used had toxic side-effects and is no longer recommended. Dextran iron, which is the preparation of choice for intravenous use, contains 50 mg iron/ml. A test dose of 1 ml should first be given, followed by doses of 100 mg (2 ml) daily on alternate days. The total dose is calculated from the following formula:

150 mg for each g/100 ml of haemoglobin deficiency

plus

1,000 mg to replace the body stores

An alternative method which is gaining favour is to give the total iron required in an intravenous infusion. It should not be used if the patient has a history of an allergic disorder. A dextran iron preparation in the appropriate dose is diluted with saline so that the solution does not contain more than 25 ml/500 ml of saline and infused; at first slowly (15–20 drops) for half an hour as a 'test period' and subsequently at an increased rate of 40 drops per minute. Reactions are few and the incidence of those due to unrecognized allergy may be reduced by prior treatment with an antihistamine drug.

Further reading

AMERICAN MEDICAL ASSOCIATION, COMMITTEE ON IRON DEFICIENCY (1968). Iron deficiency in the United States. *J. Amer. med. Ass.* **203**, 407–12.

CHARLTON, R. W. and BOTHWELL, T. H. (1970). Iron deficiency anaemia. *Semin. Hemat.* **7**, 67–85.

5 Folate and cobalamin deficiency (megaloblastic) anaemia

Introduction

Folate and cobalamin (vitamin B_{12}) coenzymes are necessary for normal cellular metabolism and are of particular importance in haemopoiesis. Severe deficiency of either B_{12} or folate leads to a derangement of DNA synthesis which is seen as the megaloblastic state in the rapidly dividing tissue of the haemopoietic system and gastrointestinal tract. The chromosomes of these cells may show morphological abnormalities and the DNA synthetic (S) and the second resting (G_2) phases of the cell cycle are prolonged. The abnormal red cell precursors in the marrow, the megaloblasts, give rise to macrocytes in the peripheral blood. Changes in the leucocytes and platelets and their precursors are also frequently present. The term macrocytic anaemia, which is sometimes used for these anaemias, is best avoided since macrocytes may be present in the blood of patients with other anaemias not associated with a megaloblastic bone marrow; for example, in the macronormoblastic reaction following haemorrhage or haemolysis. The term megaloblastic anaemia is frequently used but should, strictly speaking, be used only for those cases in which megaloblasts have been demonstrated in the bone marrow. With the availability of serum folate and vitamin B_{12} assays, bone marrow examinations are performed less frequently and the diagnosis may rest on a lowered serum vitamin level and a typical blood picture. For these reasons the term folate and/or cobalamin deficiency anaemia is preferred.

Metabolism

Vitamin B_{12} metabolism

Vitamin B_{12}, a corrinoid compound which contains cobalt, is related to a number of natural and synthetic analogues called cobalamins. These differ in the ligand attached to the cobalt atom and are interconvertible. For example, cyanocobalamin (CN ligand) is converted to hydroxycobalamin (OH ligand) on exposure to light. Several physiological coenzymes contain vitamin B_{12}.

The cobalamins are synthesized in nature by micro-organisms and are present mainly in meat and dairy products, usually attached to peptides. The daily intake in normal people varies from 1 to 5 μg, with an average daily requirement of 1 μg. Vitamin B_{12} is released from peptide linkage by gastric juice and other gastric and small-intestinal enzymes. It then combines with a glycoprotein called intrinsic factor (IF) which is secreted by the gastric parietal cells. The vitamin B_{12}–IF complex passes down to the ileum, where it is absorbed. The intrinsic factor permits attachment of the vitamin B_{12}–IF complex to the mucosal brush border but is released during absorption which also requires calcium ions and is enhanced at a pH greater than 5·6.

The absorbed vitamin B_{12} is carried into the portal blood and thence to the systemic circulation bound to a β-globulin, transcobalamin (transcorrin) II, which rapidly gives up the vitamin to the liver and other tissues. A second vitamin-B_{12}-binding protein, transcobalamin I, acts principally as a storage form of B_{12}. It is produced by granulocytic white cells and is the cause of the raised vitamin B_{12} levels found in some myeloproliferative syndromes. Recently a further protein, transcobalamin III, has been discovered, although its role has not yet been clarified. Vitamin B_{12} is excreted in the urine as well as in the bile and an enterohepatic circulation exists, due to reattachment to IF in the bowel lumen.

The complete role of cobalamin coenzymes in intermediary metabolism has not yet been worked out. One important reaction, however, is the methylation of homocysteine to methionine which requires a cobalamin coenzyme and 5-methyltetrahydrofolate (Fig. 5.1). Lack of vitamin B_{12} interferes with this reaction, leading to an accumulation of 5-methyltetrahydrofolate (the 'methyltetrahydrofolate trap') and with the regeneration of tetrahydrofolate. As a result, other folate coenzymes become depleted, inhibiting thymidylate and DNA synthesis. This may be the common pathway by which both folate and cobalamin deficiencies lead to megaloblastosis.

Another important coenzyme reaction is the conversion of methylmalonyl coenzyme A to succinyl coenzyme A so that in vitamin B_{12} deficiency there is increased urinary excretion of methylmalonic acid which can be potentiated by valine loading (Fig. 5.2). The increased blood levels of methylmalonate were once thought to be the direct cause of the neurological lesions sometimes found in vitamin B_{12} deficiency; it now seems possible that methylmalonyl CoA might inhibit the production of lipoprotein needed for myelin sheaths. However, similar neurological findings do not occur in the rare disease of congenital methylmalonic aciduria.

Folate metabolism

Folate is the name given to pteroylglutamic (folic) acid and related compounds. Food does not contain free folic acid but reduced polyglutamate derivatives, of which pteroylheptaglutamic acid is the most important (Fig. 5.3). The principal dietary sources are green vegetables, liver, milk, yeast and nuts. Considerable amounts of food folate may be destroyed in

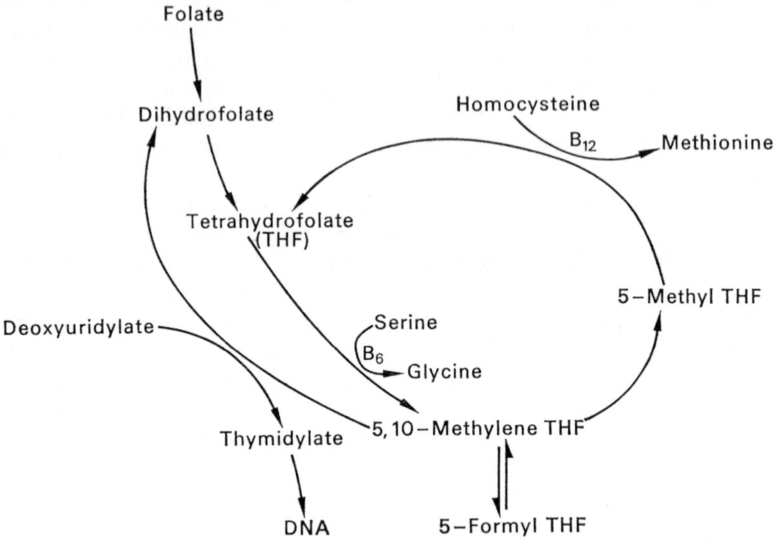

Fig. 5.1. The metabolic interrelationship of vitamin B_{12} and folate.

cooking or discarded in the cooking water. The mean daily requirement is 50–100 μg, which is increased in infancy and in pregnancy; the usual daily intake on a Western diet is 500–800 μg.

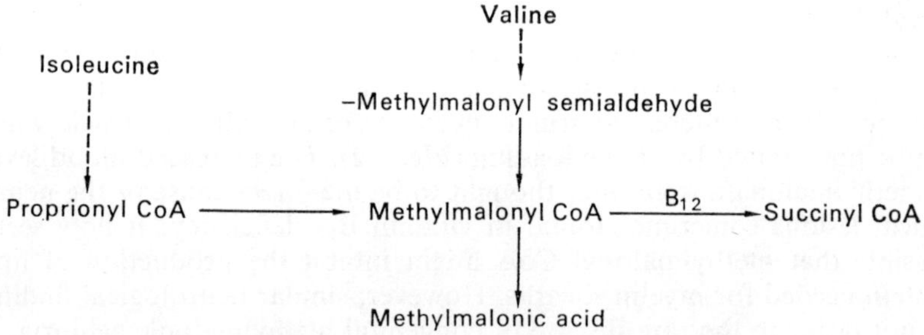

Fig. 5.2. Methylmalonic acid and vitamin B_{12}.

Folates are absorbed after deconjugation in the small intestine, mainly in the jejunum, and carried in plasma bound to protein, mostly in methyltetrahydrofolate form. The transfer to the tissues is rapid, about one-third of the body stores being in the liver, again largely as methyltetrahydrofolate. When folate intake is low, body stores will be completely depleted in 3–4 weeks, both by catabolism and by excretion into the bile and urine.

Folates function as coenzymes in the reduced tetrahydrofolate form in mammalian cell systems, accepting and transferring one carbon fragments

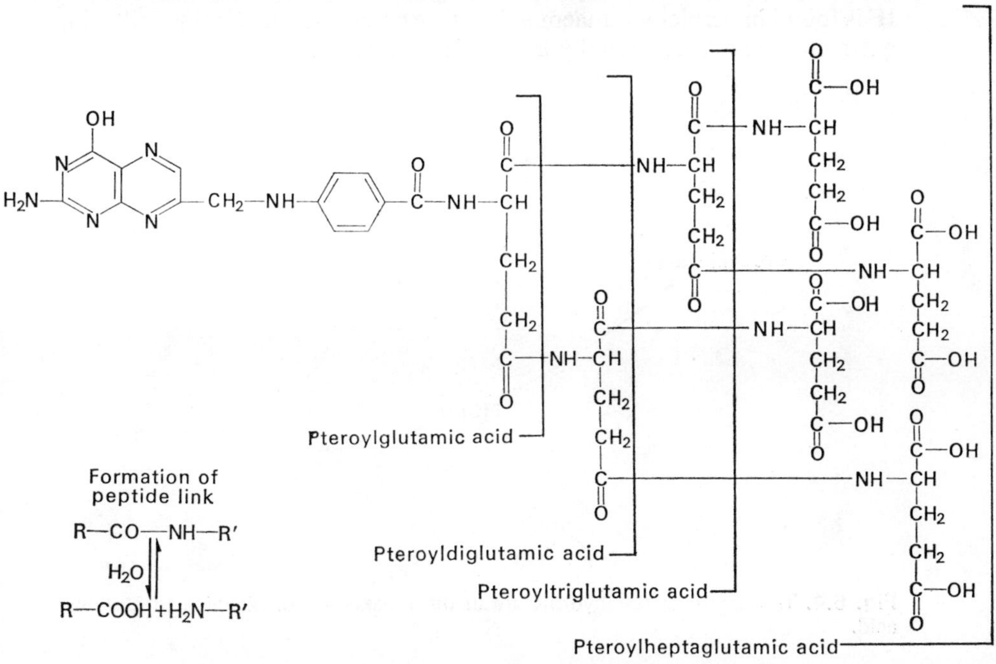

Fig. 5.3. Synthetic and natural pteroylglutamates.

needed for purine and pyrimidine synthesis. In the reduction of folic acid (see Fig. 5.1), first dihydrofolate is formed and then tetrahydrofolate; both these reactions are catalysed by dihydrofolate reductase although the latter reaction occurs much more rapidly. Another coenzyme, 5-formimino tetrahydrofolic acid, is formed from formimino glutamic acid (FIGLU), an intermediate in histidine metabolism and tetrahydrofolate. The formyl unit is utilized in the synthesis of formyl glycinamide and formyl amino-imidazolecarboxamide which are purine precursors (Fig. 5.4).

Pathogenesis

Cobalamin deficiency

Dietary deficiencies are rare and usually occur only in strict vegetarians (vegans) and other food faddists.

Intrinsic factor

Intrinsic factor deficiency leads to poor absorption and, if this is severe and prolonged, the reserves of cobalamin in the body will become depleted. The time required for this to take place and for anaemia to develop is variable, but in a previously replete person it is about 3–7 years. Lack of IF is found in pernicious anaemia, in a rare congenital deficiency, following gastrectomy and occasionally in gastric carcinoma.

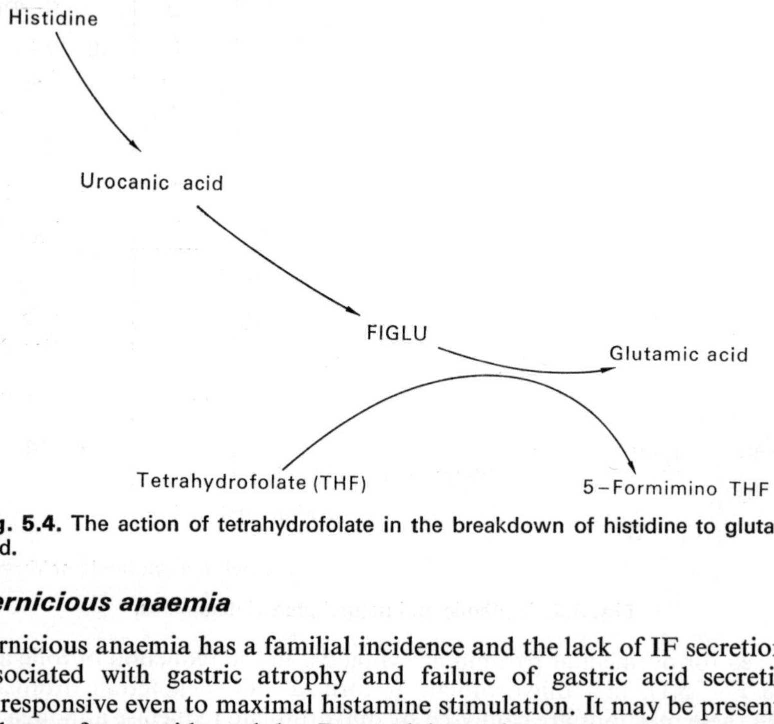

Fig. 5.4. The action of tetrahydrofolate in the breakdown of histidine to glutamic acid.

Pernicious anaemia

Pernicious anaemia has a familial incidence and the lack of IF secretion is associated with gastric atrophy and failure of gastric acid secretion, unresponsive even to maximal histamine stimulation. It may be present in a latent form evidenced by B_{12} malabsorption and a lowered serum cobalamin level for many years before it becomes manifest. The exact cause of the gastric atrophy is unknown but recently it has been suggested that it may be due to autoimmune gastritis. Nearly all patients have circulating antibodies to parietal cells and about half have antibodies to IF. The deficiency can be corrected by giving hog or human IF; this is of value in diagnosis but is not a practical form of therapy.

Congenital deficiency of IF

A congenital deficiency of IF with normal gastric acid secretion is a rare cause of a familial megaloblastic anaemia occurring in childhood (this is sometimes called pernicious anaemia of childhood, a term to be avoided). This group must be distinguished from true pernicious anaemia occurring at an early age (usually in the second decade) where gastric atrophy, achlorhydria and, often, serum antibodies are present. This latter group has a high incidence of associated endocrine disease (hypothyroidism, hypoparathyroidism, adrenocortical insufficiency and diabetes mellitus). In pernicious anaemia occurring in middle or old age there is a higher than expected incidence of associated endocrinopathy, though not so striking as in pernicious anaemia occurring at an early age.

Gastrectomy

Gastrectomy leads to a variable loss of IF, depending upon the number of parietal cells removed. Usually some years elapse before deficiency of cobalamin becomes evident since generally there are considerable cobalamin reserves in the liver and other tissues.

Gastric carcinoma

Gastric carcinoma may lead to intrinsic factor deficiency but a megaloblastic anaemia is uncommon because patients with this disorder rarely live long enough for their cobalamin reserves to be exhausted. Anaemia due to IF deficiency will respond to as little as 1 μg of vitamin B_{12} given parenterally. Often a large therapeutic dose (1–10 mg) given orally will cause a response even in the absence of intrinsic factor; this is due to absorption in the upper part of the small intestine by mass action.

Intestinal lesions

Intestinal lesions may cause B_{12} malabsorption in several ways. Lesions which allow bacterial overgrowth such as blind loops, intestinal strictures, fistulae, anastomoses and jejunal diverticulosis result in bacterial competition for B_{12} and consequent deficiency. These conditions will usually respond to the use of a broad spectrum antibiotic. The fish tapeworm (*Diphyllobothrium latum*) also absorbs vitamin B_{12}, making this unavailable to the ileal receptors. About half of those harbouring the tapeworm have a lowered serum level and about 2% develop overt megaloblastic anaemia. Resection of the ileum or its involvement in disease processes such as Crohn's disease may result in malabsorption due to blocked specific ileal receptors. A rare, autosomal recessive disease presenting with megaloblastic anaemia and proteinuria in the first or second year of life due to congenital absence of receptors for B_{12}–IF complex has been described.

Pancreatic disease

Pancreatic disease, if severe, may be an occasional cause of vitamin B_{12} malabsorption and is due both to reduction in calcium ions in the ileum from calcium soap formation and to an acid intraluminal pH from pancreatic exocrine (bicarbonate) deficiency. A similar occurrence may arise with the low pH found in the Zollinger–Ellison syndrome.

Response to folic acid

Some forms of megaloblastic anaemia due primarily to cobalamin deficiency will respond to folic acid. Pernicious anaemia is an example and in this disease the blood picture can be corrected. However, folic acid should not be used in the treatment because it will not prevent the neurological complications of cobalamin deficiency such as subacute combined degeneration of the spinal cord and mental changes.

Folate deficiency

Megaloblastic anaemia due to dietary folate deficiency is sometimes found in the tropics (tropical macrocytic anaemia) and in temperate climates. Patients with mental depression and alcoholics are particularly susceptible to dietary deficiency. Alcohol also has a direct suppressant effect on erythropoiesis. Lack of absorption occurs in such conditions as post-gastrectomy syndromes, childhood and adult coeliac disease and tropical sprue. In pregnancy the increased demands made by the fetus may lead to folate deficiency and anaemia. This can be avoided by routine folic acid supplementation of 300 μg daily throughout pregnancy. Increased demands for folate due to hyperplasia of the bone marrow are also found in haemolytic anaemias, myelofibrosis, and sideroblastic anaemia. Deficiency can also occur with increased metabolic requirements of thyrotoxicosis and excessive loss of folate may result from repeated haemodialysis. Disorders of folate metabolism occur in some patients receiving drugs, particularly those used in the treatment of epilepsy, and some oral contraceptive agents have been said to interfere with folate absorption.

Anaemias primarily due to folate deficiency may respond, at least partially, to cobalamin treatment.

Other megaloblastic anaemias

Folate deficiency megaloblastic anaemia is common in pregnancy and the puerperium if folate supplementation has not been given. True pernicious anaemia in pregnancy is rare. A number of drugs have been known to result in the development of megaloblastic anaemia, either by interference with vitamin B_{12} or folate absorption or utilization; these are shown in Table 5.1. In liver disease a relatively rare megaloblastic anaemia may result from disordered folate or cobalamin metabolism. Megaloblastosis not responding to folate or vitamin B_{12} is occasionally found in ascorbic acid deficiency, in haemolytic and sideroblastic anaemias, in erythraemic myelosis and in some leukaemias.

Table 5.1. Drugs interfering with B_{12} or folate absorption or utilization

Inhibitors	*Drugs interfering with absorption*
	Folic acid
Methotrexate	Diphenylhydantoin
Pyrimethamine	Primidone
Trimethoprim	Barbiturates
Pentamidine isethionate	Oral contraceptive agents
Triamterene	Cycloserine
	Ethyl alcohol
	Vitamin B_{12}
	Para-aminosalicylic acid
	Colchicine
	Neomycin
	Metformin
	Ethyl alcohol
Blockade of nucleoprotein synthesis	
Purine antagonists (mercaptopurine, thioguanine)	
Pyrimidine antagonists (cytosine arabinoside, 5-fluorouracil)	

Clinical features

The symptoms and signs are those of a slowly developing anaemia and those of the underlying disorder.

Pernicious anaemia

Pernicious anaemia affects both sexes equally and the patients are usually middle-aged or elderly at the time of diagnosis. There may be a family history of the disease. The onset is insidious with general symptoms such as weakness, tiredness and breathlessness of slowly increasing severity. A sore tongue and feelings of numbness and tingling in the hands and feet are common. Some patients complain of diarrhoea.

On examination the patients are usually pale and may have a slightly yellow appearance. The tongue is usually smooth and angular cheilosis is frequently present. Fever and splenomegaly are features in about one-quarter of the patients. Signs of peripheral neuropathy and of subacute combined degeneration of the spinal cord are not infrequent. Optic neuritis is occasionally seen and in some cases mental disorder dominates the picture. Premature greying of fair hair and blue eyes are more common in patients with pernicious anaemia than in other persons of the same age. A haemorrhagic diathesis is present in some patients. There is a definite association between pernicious anaemia and gastric carcinoma so that a routine barium meal is advisable in all cases.

Other anaemias

Features similar to those found in pernicious anaemia are often present with other anaemias but are usually overshadowed by the primary disorder. For example, in alcoholism other evidence of malnutrition and perhaps of liver failure may be noted, and in the malabsorption syndromes steatorrhoea may be the dominant feature; anaemia in such cases is often found incidentally.

Laboratory findings

Blood

The haematological manifestations of cobalamin or folate deficiency are identical. The haemoglobin level varies from as little as 3 g/100 ml to normal. The red cells are usually macrocytic (high MCV and MCH); they are also usually normochromic (normal MCHC) but occasionally a concurrent iron deficiency gives rise to hypochromasia. If the anaemia is severe, marked anisocytosis and poikilocytosis are also present. Neutropenia is usual (less than 2,500/μl) and the neutrophils show nuclear hypersegmentation, four or more lobes being common. The platelets are often reduced in number.

In folate deficiency the serum level will be less than 2·5 ng/ml and in cobalamin deficiency the serum level is invariably less than 100 pg/ml; occasionally both are lowered. The performance of a red cell folate level is a better reflection of body folate stores.

In megaloblastosis, there is increased cell death in the marrow ('ineffective erythropoiesis') so that the indirect-reacting (unconjugated) serum bilirubin is frequently elevated and serum lactic dehydrogenase (LDH) grossly increased. Ineffective granulopoiesis causes a raised serum muramidase, the enzyme having been released from the degradation of granulocytes.

Bone marrow

Erythroid hyperplasia with megaloblastic change is invariable. Abnormalities in the white cell series with hypersegmentation of the neutrophils and the presence of giant metamyelocytes are found in most cases. There may be maturation arrest of the megakaryocytes.

Urine

In cobalamin deficiency there is an increased excretion of methyl malonate in the urine (see Fig. 5.2) and in folate deficiency there is increased excretion of products of glutamic acid metabolism, namely formiminoglutamic acid (FIGLU) and urocanic acid (see Fig. 5.4). These latter substances are intermediary products of histidine metabolism. In up to one-third of patients with B_{12} deficiency an elevated serum folate and increased urinary FIGLU are found, due to the accumulation of intermediary products consequent upon the interference with folate metabolism produced by the vitamin B_{12} deficiency.

Diagnosis

A diagnosis of folate or cobalamin deficiency anaemia which may be suggested on clinical grounds must always be confirmed by laboratory tests. A macrocytic blood picture with neutropenia, hypersegmentation of the neutrophils and thrombocytopenia, is suspicious and should lead to a bone marrow examination which will determine whether or not megaloblastosis is present. Serum should be taken for folate and cobalamin assays. Once the blood and bone marrow specimens have been collected, treatment with folic acid and cobalamin can be given; a further diagnostic point may then be sought by observing the blood for a reticulocytosis and a rise in haemoglobin level. The reticulocyte count usually reaches a peak 5–10 days after treatment has begun.

Pernicious anaemia

In pernicious anaemia, as well as the peripheral blood and bone marrow findings described above, the serum vitamin B_{12} level is low and histamine-fast achlorhydria is present. The response to vitamin B_{12} therapy is a further diagnostic feature. A vitamin B_{12} absorption test will confirm the diagnosis and is especially valuable as it is not invalidated by prior therapy. A small radioactively labelled tracer dose of cobalamin is given by mouth and absorption of the vitamin can be assessed by measuring the radioactivity of serum, urine and faeces or by surface counting over the liver. The serum level is measured 8–10 hours later and is the most satisfactory test if ^{57}Co is used and if a gamma-spectrometer is available. In patients with pernicious anaemia the serum contains less than 0·45%/l of the dose, whereas in those with normal absorption this figure is greater than 0·65%. Measurement of the urinary excretion is frequently preferred (Schilling test). If more than 15% of the dose is excreted in 48 hours, absorption is normal, whereas in pernicious anaemia less than 5% is excreted. Faecal measurements are less popular but of value in some cases.

If poor absorption is found by any of these tests then it may be repeated (part II) using an oral tracer dose of the vitamin together with hog IF. If the intrinsic factor allows absorption to take place then pernicious anaemia is diagnosed (provided gastrectomy and gastric carcinoma have been excluded). Occasional resistance to hog IF causes abnormal results in the second test. A further test using human gastric juice (part III) is then performed.

By the use of cyanocobalamin labelled with two different isotopes (^{57}Co and ^{58}Co), one free and one bound to human gastric juice, the two tests can be combined. Since the γ-ray emissions of the two isotopes differ, permitting each to be counted in the presence of the other, the ratio of the urinary excretion of one to the other is measured. If there is malabsorption of the free vitamin but absorption of the one bound to the gastric juice, then pernicious anaemia can be diagnosed with confidence. The use of human gastric juice in this test circumvents the occasional problem of resistance to hog IF.

Other cobalamin deficiency anaemias

There are similar features in other cobalamin deficiency anaemias, but free acid may be present in the gastric juice and absorption may be normal, for example, in dietary deficiencies. Other features of the underlying disorder will be present.

Folate deficiency anaemias

The blood and bone marrow findings in folate deficiency anaemias will be similar but the serum folate will be low. Free acid may be present in the gastric juice. Tests for the absorption of other substances such as fat and xylose may give abnormal results and radiographic examination after the ingestion of barium may help in the diagnosis of various malabsorption states. Gastric and intestinal biopsies are performed in some centres.

Excessive amounts of histidine metabolites, urocanic acid and FIGLU may be detected in the urine of some patients, especially after a loading dose of histidine (see Fig. 5.4).

Folic acid absorption tests can be performed but are not undertaken routinely.

Treatment

Cobalamin deficiency

Pernicious anaemia is treated with vitamin B_{12} in the form of cyano- or hydroxycobalamin which should be given by intramuscular injection, 1,000 μg three times a week until there is a good haematological response and then weekly until the blood is normal. Thereafter, 1,000 μg are given every 3 or 4 weeks. In patients with neurological complications 1,000 μg twice weekly for several months is recommended. Other cobalamin deficiency anaemias are treated similarly except that those due to dietary deficiency may be treated orally. Folic acid and multivitamin preparations should not be used in the treatment of these conditions without coincidental cobalamin therapy since neurological complications may be precipitated or worsened.

Occasionally, the patient may be so gravely ill with profound anaemia that blood transfusion is required. This is generally not needed and it is hazardous. However, a small exchange transfusion may be used, replacing the blood removed with a packed red cell transfusion. Concomitant diuretic therapy may be given but care must be taken not to precipitate hypokalaemia which has been described as a cause of sudden death during the treatment of megaloblastic anaemia.

Folate deficiency

Folate deficiency anaemias are treated with folic acid, 5 mg three times a day until there is a good haematological response and preferably until the blood is normal. Thereafter, smaller daily doses or periodic treatment should be given depending on the underlying aetiology. If malabsorption is present or if the patient is severely ill, folic acid (30 mg daily) can be given intramuscularly. Megaloblastic anaemia due to folate antagonists can be treated with folinic acid, 3 μg four times daily. This is because the folate antagonists inhibit the reduction of dihydrofolate to the functional tetrahydrofolate form of the vitamin and folinic acid (5-formyl tetrahydrofolate) circumvents this block (see Fig. 5.1).

If the pathogenesis of the anaemia is uncertain, treatment with both vitamin B_{12} and folate may be given provided a full blood count, blood for serum, vitamin B_{12} and folate estimations and a bone marrow examination have been collected. When the anaemia has been characterized, the treatment not required should be stopped.

The response to therapy

Symptomatic improvement in pernicious anaemia is rapid, with a return of appetite and a feeling of increased well-being in the next few days; other symptoms may improve more slowly. Neurological improvement may be slow and if the nervous system involvement has been prolonged it may be incomplete.

Erythropoiesis rapidly becomes normoblastic; changes can be seen in the bone marrow within a few hours and the process is usually complete within 3 days. The reticulocyte count usually begins to rise by 48 hours and reaches its nadir by 7 days. Its height depends on the severity of the anaemia and may even reach 50% in grossly anaemic patients. In some patients the haemoglobin concentration decreases slightly, due to haemodynamic changes, before rising. Response to therapy may be delayed when there is coexistent infection and metabolic disease, especially uraemia, or coincidental iron deficiency. Iron deficiency may become apparent as the patient's haemoglobin begins to rise, due to the depletion of existing iron stores in the process of erythroid regeneration; if this occurs, iron should be given (page 78).

Further reading

HOFFBRAND, A. V. (1971). The megaloblastic anaemias. In: *Recent Advances in Haematology*, 1–76. Ed. A. Goldberg and M. C. Brain. Churchill Livingstone, Edinburgh and London.

6 Miscellaneous anaemias

Introduction

In this chapter anaemias that have not been dealt with in previous chapters are considered. They include the less common deficiency anaemias, those due to bone marrow failure, those found in pregnancy and those that are secondary to some metabolic upset.

Miscellaneous deficiency anaemias

Ascorbic acid deficiency anaemia

Ascorbic acid is necessary for normal folate metabolism and also aids iron absorption. Deficiency of a degree sufficient to cause anaemia is rare. When it does occur, it is usually due to the haemorrhagic manifestations of scurvy. Megaloblastic anaemia responding to ascorbic acid has been reported but is rare.

Pyridoxine deficiency anaemia

Pyridoxine deficiency is a very rare cause of anaemia in man, if indeed it occurs at all, but some patients with sideroblastic anaemia respond to treatment with large doses of the vitamin.

Protein deficiency anaemia

Protein deficiency may result in anaemia but only as part of severe malnutrition. It is not seen in developed countries. Protein deprivation is seen in kwashiorkor, which commonly affects infants and toddlers (1–4 years of age) during the weaning period in tropical and subtropical countries. Oedema, dermatoses and infections are the usual clinical features. Anaemia is quite common and is usually due to malaria or other infection, hookworm or other infestation and lack of iron. When these are not involved it only occurs in the final stages of the disease and may be due in part to decreased physiological requirements as a result of the lean body mass as well as to the actual lack of dietary protein. A similar anaemia may be found in the calorie protein deficiency disorder, marasmus, which is found more particularly in children under 1 year of age.

Riboflavine deficiency anaemia

Induced riboflavine deficiency can cause anaemia in man associated with a selective hypoplasia of the erythroid series in the bone marrow. Natural deficiency is rare but cases of erythroid hypoplasia in kwashiorkor sometimes respond to riboflavine (5 mg daily by injection).

Vitamin E deficiency anaemia

In premature infants fed on vitamin E deficient formulas, haemolytic anaemia may rarely develop which responds to therapy with vitamin E (tocopherol). In a few instances, anaemia in patients with kwashiorkor has been said to respond to tocopherol therapy.

Aplastic anaemia

Primary aplastic and hypoplastic anaemias

Primary aplastic anaemia is characterized by a reduction in the total amount of erythroid tissue; complete absence (aplastic anaemia) is the more severe form but lesser grades of hypoplasia are seen. There is usually an accompanying hypoplasia of the granulocytes (neutropenia) and megakaryocytes and platelets (thrombocytopenia), but occasionally pure red cell aplasia is found in the bone marrow. If this aplasia is congenital the condition is called erythrogenesis imperfecta. The primary aplastic and hypoplastic conditions are diagnosed only by the exclusion of any known causative agent or disease, and form about half the total cases.

The clinical features include those of anaemia and very often there are recurrent or severe bacterial infections associated with the neutropenia. Purpura and other haemorrhagic manifestations result from the thrombocytopenia.

Treatment with haematinics is usually unsuccessful and replacement therapy with blood transfusion is required. The transfusion of 2–3 units of blood every few weeks may keep the patient alive until a spontaneous recovery occurs. Treatment with transfusions over a long period of time often becomes complicated by red cell antibody formation and the selection of compatible blood becomes more difficult. Because these anaemias are usually unresponsive to the common haematinics they are often called 'refractory anaemias'. However, since the occasional patient may show a response, folate, cobalamin, pyridoxine and ascorbic acid treatment are often tried. Corticosteroid drugs (prednisone 50–75 mg daily) and androgens (oxymetholone 50–100 mg daily) may induce a remission. In those with serious haemorrhagic manifestations from the thrombocytopenia, corticosteroid therapy will be required and platelet transfusions are often needed. Unfortunately, antibodies to platelets frequently develop, reducing the efficacy of platelet transfusions.

The prognosis is grave and only about 50% of patients recover completely; some die from thrombocytopenic haemorrhage, infections or severe anaemia and a few progress to a chronic form of the disorder. A few develop acute leukaemia.

Secondary aplastic and hypoplastic anaemias

Secondary aplastic and hypoplastic anaemias resemble the primary type but are due to drugs, chemicals or ionizing radiation. Many drugs, including chloramphenicol and those used in the treatment of epilepsy and rheumatism, have been shown to cause bone marrow depression. Since this occurs in only a small percentage of patients taking these drugs there is thought to be an individual sensitivity. Unfortunately, this cannot be predicted even if routine blood counts are carried out. For this reason such drugs should be used only if there is no suitable alternative.

Drugs designed to kill malignant cells, such as the antimetabolites and alkylating agents, also cause bone marrow depression and this frequently limits their use. This depression is usually reversible but excessive doses or too prolonged therapy may result in irreversible bone marrow aplasia.

Chemicals used occupationally, such as benzene and the insecticides benzene hexachloride and dicophane, may also cause aplastic anaemia.

Occasional patients with viral hepatitis may develop aplastic anaemia. The rare disease, paroxysmal nocturnal haemoglobinuria, may present with bone marrow aplasia (p. 65).

The clinical picture, treatment and prognosis are similar to those of the primary aplastic anaemias, the mortality being about 50%.

Primary dysplastic anaemias

Included in the group of primary dysplastic anaemias are the erythraemic myeloses and those normoblastic or megaloblastic anaemias which do not respond to the usual haematinics; one group is characterized by the presence of 'sideroblasts'.

Those that are not sideroblastic appear to be due to an unexplained 'maturation arrest'. Since none of the haematinics or hormones is effective, this group is also included in the term 'refractory anaemia'.

Sideroblastic anaemias

In the sideroblastic anaemias there is usually marrow erythroid hyperplasia. Some of the red cell precursors resemble megaloblasts and many contain a perinuclear ring of iron-staining granules in the cytoplasm. These cells are called sideroblasts and it is from them that the condition is named. On electron microscopy, these granules can be shown to lie within the mitochondria.

The red cell morphology may be either hypochromic or dimorphic. Other features found frequently include a high serum iron with an increase in the percentage saturation of iron-binding protein (transferrin), and increased plasma iron clearance with, however, poor incorporation of iron into red cells and variable shortening of red cell life span.

The sideroblastic anaemias are classified in Table 6.1. Whilst sideroblastic anaemia is mostly an acquired disorder, on rare occasions familial cases are found with an X-linked mode of inheritance, some of this latter

Table 6.1. Classification of the sideroblastic anaemias

Hereditary
  X-linked sideroblastic anaemia
Acquired
1. Primary refractory sideroblastic anaemia
2. Secondary
   (*a*) Drugs (isoniazid, cycloserine, pyrazinamide, chloramphenicol, phenacetin)
   (*b*) Toxins (ethyl alcohol, lead)
   (*c*) Certain haematological disorders (haemolytic anaemia, leukaemia, myeloma, myeloproliferative syndromes)
   (*d*) Other conditions (rheumatoid arthritis, hypothyroidism, hyperthyroidism, metastatic carcinoma, chronic renal failure)

group of patients respond to pharmacological doses of pyridoxine although usually response is, at best, partial and it is thought that the synthesis of haem is impaired at the step requiring pyridoxine as a coenzyme. The finding of increased coproporphyrin levels and normal or slightly reduced protoporphyrin levels, however, argues against a solitary defect of the pyridoxine-dependent enzyme, δ-amino-laevulinic acid (ALA) synthetase.

Acquired sideroblastic anaemia may be idiopathic (or primary), in which event it is usually refractory to therapy with pyridoxine and other haematinics. The precise biochemical defect is unknown although it is generally believed that there is a defect in haem synthesis before ALA synthesis (see Fig. 2.6). Sideroblastic anaemia is also seen as a relatively uncommon complication of many other conditions and of certain drugs. The underlying disorder here may be a haematological disease such as haemolytic anaemia, megaloblastic anaemia, leukaemia, myeloma or myeloproliferative syndromes, or it may be a non-haematological condition; for example, rheumatoid arthritis, hypothyroidism, hyperthyroidism, metastatic carcinoma or chronic renal failure. Various drugs may occasionally produce sideroblastic anaemia by interference with haem synthesis, some directly inhibiting pyridoxine. Examples are listed in Table 6.1. Lead poisoning produces reversible sideroblastic anaemia by the inhibition of haem synthesis at several levels. However, the most frequently observed reversible sideroblastic anaemia is that seen in alcoholics following prolonged periods of drinking. In these patients the sideroblastic changes rapidly reverse when drinking ceases. The majority of these individuals are also folate deficient and the interrelationship of folate metabolism and pyridoxine is shown in Fig. 5.1.

The anaemia of chronic disorders

Anaemia in metabolic disorders

Anaemia is not infrequently found in diseases such as acute and chronic infections, rheumatoid arthritis, renal disease and malignant diseases. The anaemia is usually mild to moderate in its severity, non-progressive, frequently normocytic and hypochromic with decreased serum iron, decreased iron-binding capacity and normal reticuloendothelial iron stores. It appears that there is impairment of iron release from the stores to the plasma, accounting for the iron-deficient type of erythropoiesis. In some, there may be a haemolytic element; in others, the bone marrow is actively infiltrated with abnormal cells. However, in many there is no obvious abnormality of the bone marrow. A metabolic depression of erythropoiesis has been postulated in some cases.

Anaemia in endocrine disorders

Anaemia is found in pituitary and thyroid hypofunction, probably as a result of lowered oxygen needs of the tissues. It can be reversed by thyroxine although the response is often slow.

Some refractory anaemias may be benefited by testosterone, but deficiency of this hormone is not associated with anaemia and its effect is probably anabolic. The beneficial effect of thymectomy in some cases of erythroid aplasia may have an immunological basis.

Leucoerythroblastic anaemia

In some conditions, anaemia is characterized by the presence of immature leucocytes and erythroblasts in the peripheral blood. The bone marrow is usually infiltrated with malignant cells or is the site of myelofibrosis. Other causes of such an anaemia include myelomatosis, lymphomas, leukaemias, lipid storage disorders and severe infections. The diagnosis is made by bone marrow biopsy. Treatment is directed to the underlying disorder but blood transfusions are also frequently required.

Anaemia in liver disease

Anaemia in liver disease may be due to blood loss and subsequently to iron deficiency. Macrocytic anaemia may be found with a normoblastic or a megaloblastic bone marrow. The aetiology of the normoblastic type is not fully understood and it does not respond to folate or cobalamin. Megaloblastic anaemia in liver disease is usually due to disorders of folate metabolism but may also rarely be due to disorders of cobalamin metabolism and therefore both vitamins should be given in treatment initially. Folate deficiency may follow dietary lack (especially in alcoholics), poor absorption, enzymic disturbances in the liver and increased needs following haemorrhage. Cobalamin metabolism may be upset as a result of decreased absorption and lowered stores in the liver.

Anaemia in pregnancy

Pregnancy anaemia is not a specific entity but it is worthy of separate consideration since an acutely lowered maternal haemoglobin level may be associated with fetal anoxia and death. Although there is no clear statistical evidence that chronic anaemia is an appreciable cause of high fetal loss, most obstetricians try to ensure that their patients have a normal haemoglobin concentration at term. A slightly lower than normal haemoglobin value with normochromic normocytic red cells may result from the physiological hydraemia of pregnancy. Nevertheless, all patients with haemoglobin levels below 11·5 g/100 ml should be investigated further to see if iron deficiency or folate deficiency is present. The high incidence of iron deficiency in pregnancy (see p. 75) has led to the routine issue of iron preparations to pregnant women. However, the issue of prophylactic iron does not mean that it will be taken and, if deficiency is noted late in pregnancy, a total-dose intravenous infusion of iron is often given.

Folate deficiency due to fetal demands is common but its incidence varies in different communities, as does the recommendation of the prophylactic use of folic acid tablets. A theoretical objection to its use is that it might precipitate neurological changes in the very rare patient with incipient pernicious anaemia. If given, a dose of 300–500 μg daily is adequate. This dose is insufficient to precipitate neurological symptoms in such cases. Folate deficiency may be precipitated after parturition by lactation giving rise to a postpartum megaloblastic anaemia.

Further reading

BARRETT-CONNOR, E. (1972). Anemia and infection. *Amer. J. Med.* **52**, 242–53.

BATEMAN, C. J. T. and MOLLIN, D. L. (1970). Sideroblastic anaemia. *Brit. J. Hosp. Pract.* **4**, 371–9.

SANCHEZ-MEDAL, L. (1971). The hemopoietic action of androstanes. *Progr. Hemat.* **7**, 111–36.

VAN DER WEYDEN, M. and FIRKIN, B. G. (1972). The management of aplastic anaemia in adults. *Brit. J. Haemat.* **22**, 1–7.

YUNIS, ADEL A. (1970). Drug-induced bone marrow injury. *Advanc. Intern. Med.* **15**, 357–75.

7 The myeloproliferative disorders

Introduction

An increase in the number of erythrocytes, leucocytes and thrombocytes in the peripheral blood may be physiological, reactionary or due to a myeloproliferative disorder. Erythrocytosis is considered in this chapter, leucocytosis in Chapter 8 and thrombocytosis in Chapter 11. The concept of the myeloproliferative disorders was introduced by Dameshek for those conditions in which proliferation of bone marrow cells is greater than physiological or reactive and is generally progressive. Some of these conditions are rather similar and it has been suggested that the basic defect is neoplastic proliferation of a pluripotential stem cell capable of differentiating along one or more multiple lines. They are considered to be neoplastic and may be 'benign' or 'malignant', 'chronic' or 'acute'. The chronic types are chronic granulocytic leukaemia (Chapter 9), polycythaemia vera (this chapter), myelofibrosis (this chapter) and idiopathic thrombocythaemia (Chapter 11). The myeloblastic leukaemias (Chapter 9), erythraemic myelosis (this chapter) and malignant myelofibrosis (this chapter) comprise the acute forms. The lymphoproliferative disorders include the lymphoid types of leukaemias (Chapter 9) and the lymphomas (Chapter 10). The related conditions, myeloma and macroglobulinaemia, are also considered in Chapter 9. The possible interrelationship of these disorders is illustrated in Fig. 7.1.

Erythrocytosis

An increase in the concentration of erythrocytes is called erythrocytosis. It may be relative, due to a lowered plasma volume, or absolute, due to an increase in the body red cell mass above the normal 30 ± 5 ml/kg body weight for males or 25 ± 5 ml/kg for females. The causes are classified in Table 7.1.

Relative erythrocytosis

In relative erythrocytosis there is an increased concentration of erythrocytes in the blood due to a decrease in the plasma volume. Since the leucocytes and thrombocytes may also appear increased, the term polycythaemia may be used. The total red cell is not increased, however. The low plasma volume may be due to loss of fluid externally as in burns, vomiting and diarrhoea, or internally into the tissues. It is also found in stress erythrocytosis.

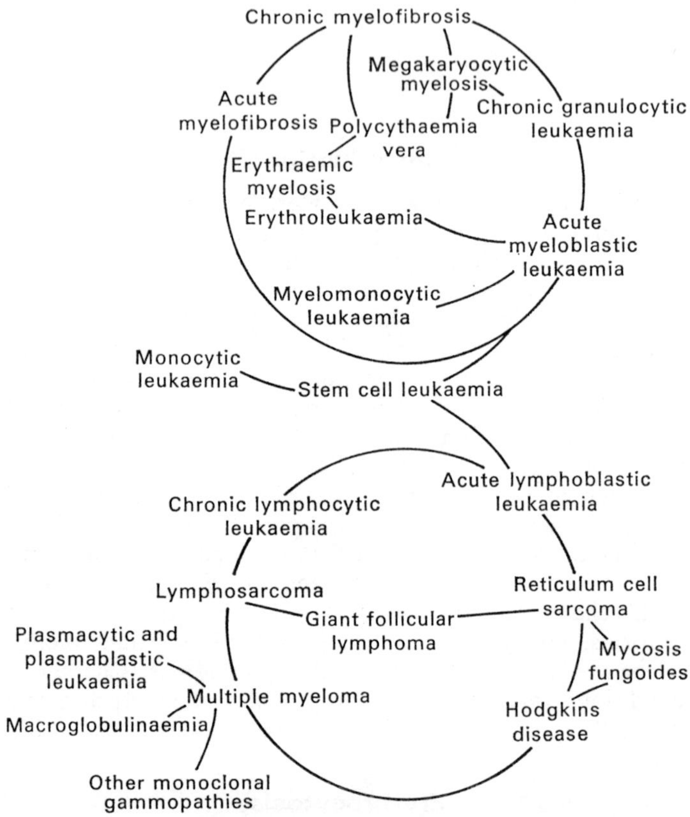

Fig. 7.1. Interrelationship of the myeloproliferative disorders.

Stress erythrocytosis

In this condition, which is poorly understood, there is a relative erythrocytosis. Patients usually have an anxiety state and clinically resemble patients with true erythrocytosis. The haematocrit is raised to between 55 and 60% or so, but the total red cell mass is normal. The cause of the lowered plasma volume is not known. The spleen is not palpable, as it often is in true erythrocytosis.

True erythrocytosis

An absolute increase in the red cell mass may occur as a primary neoplastic process in polycythaemia vera or secondary to a number of causes via the intermediacy of increased erythropoietin production, whose

Table 7.1. Classification of erythrocytosis

Relative erythrocytosis
1. Dehydration
2. Stress erythrocytosis

True erythrocytosis

A. *With increased erythropoietin levels*
1. Physiological—high altitude
2. Hypoxia
   (*a*) Cyanotic congenital heart disease
   (*b*) Pulmonary disease
   (*c*) Renal disease
   (*d*) Central nervous system disease with hypoventilation
   (*e*) Abnormal haemoglobins with increased affinity for oxygen
3. Drugs
   (*a*) Cobalt
   (*b*) Androgens, glucocorticoids, thyroxine
4. Inappropriate erythropoietin secretion by tumours

B. *With low or normal erythropoietin levels*
1. Polycythaemia vera

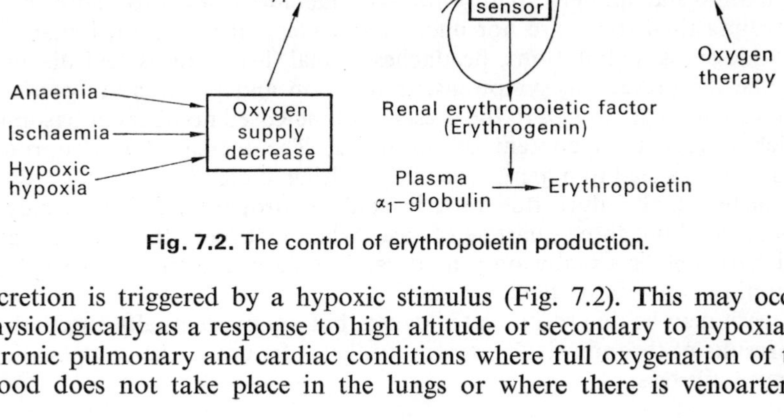

Fig. 7.2. The control of erythropoietin production.

secretion is triggered by a hypoxic stimulus (Fig. 7.2). This may occur physiologically as a response to high altitude or secondary to hypoxia in chronic pulmonary and cardiac conditions where full oxygenation of the blood does not take place in the lungs or where there is venoarterial shunting of blood. Chronic sulph- and methaemoglobinaemia may produce polycythaemia by the same mechanism. Cobalt is toxic to cell respiration and this results in compensatory erythropoietin elaboration. Androgens also stimulate erythropoietin production.

Some familial cases of polycythaemia have been found to be due to the presence of an abnormal haemoglobin which possesses an increased affinity for oxygen and results in decreased oxygen delivery to the tissues.

Secondary erythrocytosis or polycythaemia may be found in renal diseases and especially in renal carcinoma; it is thought to be due to excessive erythrogenin or erythropoietin secreted by the diseased tissue. Carcinoma of the liver, cerebellar haemangioblastoma, uterine tumours, phaeochromocytomas and Cushing's syndrome are all rare causes of secondary polycythaemia.

Erythraemia (polycythaemia vera)

In erythraemia there is a true increase in the red cell mass. An increase in leucocytes and in thrombocytes is also frequently present, hence the alternative name *polycythaemia vera.* The aetiology is not known and the disorder is generally considered to be a benign neoplasm. It is classified as one of the myeloproliferative disorders and transformation into myelofibrosis is common. Termination as acute myeloblastic leukaemia also occurs but usually only in patients treated with radioactive phosphorus.

Clinical features

It is more frequent in men than women. Symptoms develop in middle age and are usually attributable to the increased red cell mass. As a result of the increased RCV the patients appear plethoric and, because of the presence of increased amounts of reduced haemoglobin in the capillary circulation, they may appear slightly cyanosed. The high haemoglobin concentration is associated with a high blood viscosity, with consequent stagnation and liability to thrombosis. Haemorrhages, especially in the gastrointestinal tract, are not uncommon. General ill health, irritability, breathlessness, palpitations, headaches, visual disturbances and dizziness may be the presenting symptoms. Indigestion and pruritus are common and have been attributed to the presence of increased numbers of basophils which have a high content of histamine. The increased nucleoprotein turnover may lead to hyperuricaemia, resulting in secondary gout or, more seriously, renal failure due to uric acid nephropathy. Splenomegaly is present in about three-quarters of cases when first seen; the spleen is firm and hard and is usually only moderately enlarged. Pain due to splenic infarction is not infrequent.

Death may be due to unrelated causes but many eventually succumb to the results of thrombosis, haemorrhage, heart failure or the complications of myelofibrosis.

Laboratory findings

The blood is thick and viscous, making the preparation of a smear difficult. A low ESR is one result of this. The haematocrit is generally raised to between 60 and 70% and the haemoglobin concentration is 18–24 g/100 ml. The red cell count is also raised proportionately so that the erythrocytes are usually normochromic and normocytic, although microcytes are sometimes prominent. After venesection or bleeding, hypochromasia may be seen. The red cell mass may be as high as 90 ml/kg body weight.

Table 7.2. Differential diagnosis of polycythaemia

	Polycythaemia vera	*Secondary erythrocytosis*	*Stress erythrocytosis*
Haemoglobin haematocrit	Raised +++	Raised ++	Raised +
White cell count	Raised ++→+++	Normal	Normal
Platelet count	Raised +→+++	Normal	Normal
Splenomegaly	In 70%	No	No
Bone marrow	Generalized hyperplasia	Erythroid hyperplasia	Normal
Red cell mass	Raised +++	Raised ++	Normal
Plasma volume	Usually normal	Usually normal	Low

The leucocyte count is usually raised, often to 30,000/μl and occasionally up to 70,000/μl. Most of the increase is in the neutrophil granulocytes which show a 'shift to the left' (or increase in more primitive forms).

The platelet count is frequently raised above normal and megakaryocytic fragments may occasionally be found in the blood smears. Sometimes the laboratory findings merge with those of myelofibrosis or idiopathic thrombocythaemia. The bleeding time may be prolonged due to congestion in the capillaries and to functional abnormalities of the platelets.

The bone marrow shows a generalized hyperplasia, frequently with absent reticuloendothelial iron stores since bleeding is so common.

Diagnosis

The diagnosis is made on the clinical examination and on the blood findings (see Table 7.1). Underlying disorders which give rise to secondary polycythaemia should be excluded as far as possible (Table 7.2). The increase in the red cell mass should be measured using the radiochromium labelling technique.

Treatment

Venesection of 500 ml of blood may be beneficial as a preliminary treatment to alleviate symptoms. It can be repeated to further reduce the red cell mass and induce iron deficiency anaemia. However, since it has no effect on the increased numbers of platelets, more definitive treatment is recommended. This is aimed at depressing the bone marrow and is best accomplished with radioactive phosphorus. This generally causes a reduction in the red cell mass in 6–8 weeks' time, and the remission may last from 6 months to several years. A reduction in the platelet count also occurs. Its use is associated with a slightly increased risk of developing acute leukaemia but the over-all survival of patients treated with radioactive phosphorus is similar to that of other treatments.

Chemotherapy with busulphan or other cytotoxic drugs is sometimes used as an alternative. The aim of chemotherapy is to ameliorate symptoms and to keep the haematocrit in the region of 40–45%.

Because of the frequency with which hyperuricaemia occurs, the serum uric acid should be determined before therapy is begun. The cell destruction brought about by cytotoxic therapy results in further elevation of the uric acid level. This can be controlled with the xanthine oxidase inhibitor, allopurinol, in a dose of 100 mg three times daily.

Erythraemic myelosis

Malignant disorders of the erythroid tissues, which may be acute or chronic, are included under the general heading of erythraemic myelosis. The erythroid tissues show hyperplasia and dysplasia. Nucleated red cells are often found in the peripheral blood and there is usually an associated anaemia.

Acute erythraemic myelosis

Acute erythraemic myelosis is also called Di Guglielmo's disease; clinically it closely resembles acute leukaemia.

The blood usually shows a normochromic normocytic anaemia. Nucleated red cells are usually present although reticulocytosis is not common. The leucocyte count is generally low and in some cases abnormal leucocytes are seen. Thrombocytopenia is usual.

The diagnosis is usually made upon examination of the bone marrow. Erythroid hyperplasia is marked and there are many abnormal cells present. Giant and fragmented nuclei are common; many abnormal mitotic figures may be seen. Often megaloblastic cells are present but the disorder does not respond to vitamin B_{12} or folic acid therapy. The abnormal nucleated erythroid cells often show clumps of positive material when the periodic acid–Schiff (PAS) stain is used. Increased numbers of myeloblasts may be present in the marrow and the condition frequently progresses to an acute myeloblastic leukaemia.

Chemotherapy is generally ineffective but mercaptopurine should be tried. Symptomatic treatments, including blood transfusions, are given.

Erythroleukaemia

This name is given to a concomitant malignant proliferation of both erythroid and granulocytic cells; if the patient survives long enough the leukaemic element usually predominates.

Chronic erythraemic myelosis

Some patients with abnormal erythroid precursors in their bone marrow pursue a chronic course similar to that of the hypoplastic anaemias. The condition resembles idiopathic sideroblastic anaemia which should be excluded before the diagnosis is accepted. There is no specific treatment, but symptomatic treatment with blood transfusions may allow the patients to survive for several years.

Myelofibrosis

Introduction

Myelofibrosis is known by many other names, including myeloid metaplasia and myelosclerosis. It is one of the myeloproliferative disorders in which the haemopoietic bone marrow is gradually replaced by fibroblastic proliferation. Myeloid metaplasia in the liver and spleen and other organs occurs and may precede marrow fibrosis, suggesting that it occurs primarily rather than as a result of the marrow disorder. The condition is relatively uncommon and occurs in middle and late life.

Clinical features

Clinically, the patient often presents with symptoms of anaemia. Splenomegaly is prominent and may be first noticed by the patient; pain may be felt in the spleen itself or may be due to pressure effects on other tissues. For example, pressure on the stomach may cause early satiety when food is ingested. The liver may be enlarged and signs of hypermetabolism such as weight loss and fever may be present.

As with the other myeloproliferative syndromes, hyperuricaemia may be present, causing attacks of gout or uric acid nephropathy.

Laboratory findings

Anaemia and leucoerythroblastosis are usually present. The erythrocytes show anisocytosis, teardrop poikilocytosis and polychromasia; normoblasts are present. The leucocyte count varies from below normal up to 20,000 or 30,000 cells/μl. A small proportion of the leucocytes are myeloblasts; myelocytes are also present, together with normal segmented neutrophils. Occasionally, the picture merges with that of granulocytic leukaemia. The thrombocytes are often increased in numbers; giant and other abnormal forms may be seen in the film. Thrombocytopenia may be present in the later stages.

Bone marrow is difficult to aspirate and the attempt often results in a 'dry' or 'blood' tap. Trephine biopsy reveals an increase in reticular fibres and fibroblastic proliferation, the infiltrate often being very cellular. The megakaryocytes are usually abnormal with an increase in average size and a bizarre nuclear configuration.

Splenic puncture aspirates reveal myeloid metaplasia, the smears containing normoblasts, myelocytes and megakaryocytes.

X-ray examination may show some increased density of the bones in about one-third of cases.

Diagnosis

The diagnosis is established with certainty only by bone marrow biopsy but the presence of a leucoerythroblastic anaemia, dry marrow tap and positive splenic puncture is highly suggestive. Secondary disorders of the bone marrow, such as infiltration by carcinoma cells or lipid storage cells, myelomatosis, leukaemias and lymphomas may give a similar picture.

Occasionally, the disease may be confused with chronic granulocytic leukaemia but the presence of the Philadelphia chromosome in the latter condition will distinguish the two (p. 130).

Treatment and course

Symptoms which may require treatment include those due to anaemia, those due to the enlarged spleen and those due to infections.

Anaemia is usually treated with blood transfusions; anabolic and corticosteroid hormones may also help. In some patients splenectomy is beneficial since, in addition to producing red cells, the enlarged spleen may increase haemolysis and inhibit erythropoiesis in some sites. The liver frequently enlarges following splenectomy. In some patients removal of the spleen is definitely harmful since effective erythropoietic tissue is lost. An attempt is made to predict the effects of such an operation by combined radioactive iron and chromium study in order to assess the relative erythropoietic activity of the bone marrow and the spleen and the degree to which sequestration of red cells is occurring in the spleen. If hypersplenism rather than bone marrow failure is playing the dominant role, then chemotherapy with busulphan or radiotherapy may have some effect. Infections are treated along the usual lines; haemorrhagic complications are usually due to thrombocytopenia from marrow failure and may be ameliorated using corticosteroid therapy. Due to the chronicity of the process and antibody formation from repeated blood transfusions, platelet transfusions are usually not a practical measure.

The serum uric acid should be measured and significant hyperuricaemia can usually be controlled with allopurinol (100 mg three times daily).

The disease takes a very variable course, from death within a month or so (malignant myelofibrosis) to a relatively benign disease lasting many years.

Further reading

DAMESHEK, W. and GUNZ, F. (1964). Leukaemia and the myeloproliferative disorders. In: *Leukaemia*, 356–402. Grune and Stratton, New York.

PANEL DISCUSSION (1968). The treatment of polycythaemia. *Blood* **32**, 483–506.

8 Leucopoiesis and its disorders

Introduction

The leucocytes found in the blood and tissues of the body are derived from precursor cells in the bone marrow, spleen, lymph nodes and other reticular tissues by a process of multiplication and maturation. The factors which control leucopoiesis and the distribution of the mature cells between the blood and the tissues are not fully understood and probably differ for each cell series. For this reason and because of the differences of function, the granulocytes, lymphocytes and monocytes are usually considered separately. First, however, the leucocytes as a whole are considered. Those circulating in the blood form only a small proportion (less than 1 %) of the total and whilst they usually reflect changes in the tissue leucocytes, this is not always so. The normal values for the concentration of all the leucocytes in the blood of adults is 4,000–10,000/μl. A small proportion of healthy adults have figures outside this range and the concentration is higher in babies. The numbers of each cell type are usually calculated from the differential leucocyte count and it will be remembered that at birth neutrophils predominate, but that from the second week of life to the second year the lymphocytes are the most frequent cells. These then show a gradual relative decline to adult levels when the neutrophils are usually, but not always, preponderant.

An increase in the concentration of leucocytes in the peripheral blood is called leucocytosis; it may be due to granulocytosis (neutrophilia, eosinophilia or basophilia), lymphocytosis or monocytosis.

A decrease is called leucopenia and may be due to granulocytopenia (neutropenia, eosinopenia or basopenia), lymphopenia or monocytopenia.

Normal leucopoiesis

Granulopoiesis

Granulocytes are produced by maturation of precursor (stem) cells in the bone marrow (see Fig. 1.4). The myeloblast is the first recognizable cell of the series. This matures into promyelocytes and myelocytes which multiply (the mitotic pool) and then mature as post-mitotic cells into metamyelocytes, stab cells and segmented granulocytes. This forms the marrow granulocyte reserve pool. The three different types—neutrophils, eosinophils and basophils—can be recognized at the myelocyte stage.

Neutrophil granulocytes

It has been estimated that an adult has 3×10^{12} granulocytes and, of these, less than 1% (about 20,000 million) are in the peripheral blood. The bone marrow contains 900 g, the other tissues 600 g and the blood 10 g of granulocytes. Most of the cells in the marrow and tissues are mature and constitute a reserve which is mobilized during infection. Cell factors which influence the multiplication, maturation and release of cells from the marrow are not known but the granulocytes themselves contain a leucocytosis-inducing factor (LIF) which is released from the dead cells. This appears to stimulate both the release of reserves and the production of new granulocytes. The removal or loss of cells from the circulating granulocyte pool may also stimulate granulocyte mobilization. In addition, the spleen plays some part in the control of circulating granulocytes since after splenectomy there is an increase in the number of cells in the blood. Corticotrophin injections cause a neutrophil leucocytosis and the adrenal corticosteroids may have a physiological role in leucopoiesis. The life cycle of neutrophil leucocytes has been estimated by a variety of radioisotopic methods with varying results. The time from mitosis to maturation is probably about 3 or 4 days. Once released into the circulation the mean intravascular life has been estimated at 6–20 hours. In the blood the granulocytes are distributed equally between a circulating pool and a marginating pool. They can pass freely into the tissues and may be lost in the saliva and intestinal secretions or destroyed in the blood or in the tissues. The total life span of the granulocyte, particularly after leaving the blood, is unknown. They cannot return to the blood stream.

The function of the neutrophil granulocyte is the defence of the body against infections. Cells migrate to areas of infection (chemotaxis) and, by phagocytosis, ingest certain types of invading bacteria. Mobilization of reserves occurs and the area becomes crowded with granulocytes; this is reflected in the neutrophilia in the blood.

A number of chemotactic factors have been described, including bacterial products, tissue proteases and a complex of the fifth, sixth and seventh components of complement. Next, the material to be ingested is changed in such a way as to allow phagocytosis to occur. This is called opsonization (or opsonification) and depends upon the presence of antibody, complement and other heat-labile factors. Opsonized micro-organisms then attach to receptor sites on the cell membrane and are phagocytosed and destroyed.

Eosinophil granulocytes

Eosinophil granulocytes are present in the blood, bone marrow and other tissues. Eosinophils are formed in the marrow but the factors influencing their multiplication, maturation and release are not fully understood. They may be produced in the bone marrow in response to an antigen and this process can be divided into two phases, the inductive and the proliferative. There is a relationship between the thymus-processed (T) lymphocytes (see below) and eosinophils since the inductive phase is stopped by experimental T-cell depletion or by anti-lymphocyte serum (which works against T cells). The proliferative phase, which follows some 24 hours later and results in a great increase in eosinophils, is not inhibited by anti-lymphocyte serum but is prevented by cytotoxic drugs. The exact nature of antigen, antibody, complement and activated lymphocyte interactions leading to eosinophilia remains speculative.

Eosinophils are mildly phagocytic but do not play a direct part in the defence against bacterial invasion. They are frequently associated with allergic reaction.

Basophil granulocytes

Basophil granulocytes contain histamine but their precise role in physiology is uncertain. They are not phagocytic but may play a role in immunity by releasing histamine at sites of inflammation.

Lymphopoiesis

Lymphocytes are produced by maturation from lymphoblasts in the lymphatic tissues of the body. An intermediate prolymphocyte stage is recognized by some authors and the mature cells are of two types, the large and the small. Some consider that the large lymphocyte is the precursor of the small; others think that they develop independently.

It has been estimated that there are 6×10^{12} lymphocytes in the body; of these 0·2% (12×10^9) are present in the peripheral blood. The blood contains 3 g, the bone marrow 100 g, the spleen and lymphatic tissues 100 g and the other tissues 1,300 g.

Factors influencing the multiplication, maturation and release of cells from the lymphatic tissues are poorly understood.

There appear to be two populations of lymphocytes, the thymus-derived antigen-reactive T cells and the non-thymus-derived antibody-forming precursor B cells. Thus lymphocytes are derived from stem cells which have migrated to the primary lymphoepithelial organs, either the thymus (T) or to the human equivalent of the bursa of Fabricus (B).

Once lymphocytes have been generated in these primary lymphoid organs they migrate to the secondary lymphoid organs such as the lymph nodes and spleen. The thymus-derived small lymphocytes (T cells) are long-lived cells which recirculate and populate the paracortical areas of the lymph nodes, whilst the thymic-independent lymphocytes (B cells) populate the follicles and medullary cords of the lymph nodes.

The main function of lymphocytes is immunological. In contrast to that in the primary lymphoid organs, lymphocyte proliferation and differentiation in the secondary lymphoid tissues is antigen dependent. Antigen stimulates B cells to change to plasma cells and secrete antibody immunoglobulin. On the other hand, T cells respond to antigen by eventually forming sensitized small lymphocytes which are involved in cellular immunity (including delayed hypersensitivity and graft-versus-host reactions). Soluble products (lymphokines) may be produced and contribute to these reactions.

Plasmacytopoiesis

The plasma cells (plasmacytes) are produced by maturation of plasmablasts and proplasmacytes in the reticular tissues of the body. Normally, relatively few (comprising less than 0·5% of the leucocytes) are present in the peripheral blood and they are not commonly recognized in ordinary blood smears. They can be found in white cell concentrates and an occasional proplasmacyte, sometimes in mitosis, may also be seen. Plasma cells are concerned with antibody formation (see above).

Monocytopoiesis

The monocytes are derived from the reticular tissue of the bone marrow and other organs such as the liver and spleen. They are produced by maturation of monoblasts and promonocytes. They are normally present in the blood in a concentration of 200–800/μl. It has been estimated that blood contains about 500,000 and there must be many more in the tissues. Their life cycle is unknown. They phagocytose foreign bodies and debris and are associated with chronic inflammation.

Disorders of leucopoiesis

Disorders of leucopoiesis are usually reflected by changes in the peripheral blood. Excessive numbers (leucocytosis) may be present due to physiological or pathological disturbances which upset the balance between production, storage and distribution of the leucocytes. Two types of pathological leucocytosis may be distinguished, the reactive and the leukaemic. A reactive type follows known stimuli and regresses if the stimulus is removed. The leukaemic type is part of a progressive malignant proliferation of the leucopoietic tissues of uncertain aetiology (p. 121).

Decreased numbers of leucocytes in the blood (leucopenia) are always pathological and most frequently affect the neutrophils. The disorders of the different leucocyte types are discussed separately.

Neutrophil leucocytosis (neutrophilia)

Physiological

Normal variations occur around the usual neutrophil concentration of 2,500–7,500/μl of blood. Lower and higher levels are occasionally found in healthy subjects, and tropical Africans often have relatively low levels. Variations may occur at different times of the day, usually with higher values in the afternoon. A physiological leucocytosis may also be found following exercise, during pregnancy and during childbirth.

Reactive

A neutrophil leucocytosis with counts of 10,000–50,000/μl may be found as a reaction in a variety of conditions. A leucocytosis-promoting factor can be isolated from inflammatory exudates, and infections (especially those due to pyogenic bacteria) are usually associated with leucocytosis. Tissue necrosis (for example, in coronary thrombosis or other infarctions and following burns and trauma) and blood loss due to haemorrhage and haemolysis cause a leucocytosis, as do malignant neoplasms, especially if they are associated with necrosis. Pathological exercise (for example, in epileptic fits) is a further cause. A similar mechanism may cause leucocytosis in paroxysmal tachycardia.

As well as the increased concentration of neutrophils, there is a relatively greater proportion of young forms and a few myelocytes may be found in the peripheral blood. This change is called 'a shift to the left'. Occasionally very high counts, up to 150,000 neutrophils/μl, and a more marked shift to the left are found. The resulting blood picture resembles that of chronic granulocytic leukaemia and is called a leukaemoid reaction. The alkaline phosphatase test is helpful in differentiating the two (p. 131).

Leukaemic

The myeloproliferative disorders, chronic granulocytic leukaemia, myelofibrosis and polycythaemia vera, are associated with a leucocytosis and a shift to the left. A neutrophil leucocytosis with cell counts usually above 50,000/μl occurs in a rare form of chronic granulocytic leukaemia, in which most of the circulating cells are of mature morphology. This variant is called *neutrophilic leukaemia.*

Eosinophil leucocytosis (eosinophilia)

Eosinophil leucocytosis is an increase in the number of eosinophils in the blood above 400 cells/μl. (A direct eosinophil count using a Fuchs–Rosenthal chamber and a special diluting fluid containing eosin and acetone is more accurate than a count based on the total differential leucocyte count but in practice the latter often suffices.)

Eosinophilia occurs in allergic disorders such as asthma, in parasitic infestations, in various skin diseases, in some neoplasms such as disseminated carcinomatosis and in about 15% of cases of Hodgkin's disease. It has been shown that eosinophilia and the specific anti-parasite immune reaction are separable phenomena and may indicate that different antigens are activating different parts of the host's immune mechanism. Increases are also found in some cases of polyarteritis nodosa and pulmonary eosinophilia.

Leukaemic eosinophil leucocytosis occurs as part of a chronic granulocytic leukaemia and a very rare eosinophilic leukaemia has also been described.

Basophil leucocytosis (basophilia)

Basophil leucocytosis is an increase in the number of basophils above 100/μl. It is rare, being found in some leukaemias and pre-leukaemias.

Lymphocytosis

A reactive lymphocytosis of more than 3,000 cells/μl is found in a variety of infections, especially in those due to viruses (varicella, rubella and mumps), pertussis, brucellosis, salmonellosis, tuberculosis and syphilis. Two infections associated with a marked lymphocytosis are especially important as they may be confused with leukaemia. They are infectious lymphocytosis and infectious mononucleosis (p. 116). A leukaemic lymphocytosis is found in lymphocytic leukaemia and in some cases of lymphosarcoma.

Plasmacytosis

A reactive plasmacytosis occurs in various virus infections such as rubella and infectious mononucleosis. Leukaemic plasmacytosis occurs in an unusual form of multiple myeloma called *plasma cell leukaemia* (p. 136).

Monocytosis

A reactive monocytosis of over 800 monocytes/μl is found in a variety of infections, usually chronic in nature. They include salmonellosis (enteric fevers), tuberculosis, brucellosis and subacute bacterial endocarditis. Protozoal (malaria, kala-azar and trypanosomiasis) and rickettsial infections may also be associated with a monocytosis. It is also common in infectious mononucleosis.

A leukaemic monocytosis is found in monocytic leukaemia and in some forms of granulocytic leukaemia. Monocytes may also be prominent in the blood of patients with Hodgkin's disease and other malignant reticuloses.

Infectious mononucleosis

Infectious mononucleosis, which is frequently called glandular fever, is an acute infection characterized by lymphadenopathy, the appearance of atypical lymphocytes in the blood and by a positive heterophil antibody test. Recent studies have indicated that a member of the herpes group of viruses, the Epstein–Barr (EB) virus, is associated with the disease although it has not yet been conclusively shown to be the causative agent. It is possible that the virus is a 'passenger', although EB virus only replicates in the cells of the lymphoreticular system and the virus will stimulate, in tissue culture, leucocytes of infectious mononucleosis patients to proliferate into blastoid cells harbouring the virus.

Clinical

The condition may be asymptomatic, but usually there is generalized malaise, a sore throat, headache, muscular aches and fever. The superficial lymph nodes and especially those of the posterior triangle of the neck are enlarged, often there is an exanthematous skin rash and moderate splenomegaly is found in about half the cases. Occasionally, the spleen ruptures. Petechiae may be seen, especially on the soft palate. Pharyngeal infection and tonsillar enlargement with an exudate and sometimes a membrane are seen. In a few cases jaundice develops and the condition may closely resemble infectious hepatitis. Rarely, there is evidence of nervous system involvement. Infectivity is low but outbreaks may occur in closed communities and it is especially common in colleges and universities where it is thought to be transmitted by deep kissing.

Blood picture

A neutrophil leucocytosis may be found in the early stages, but this is soon replaced by a lymphocytosis with a relative or absolute neutropenia. Typically, the lymphocyte count is in the 5,000–15,000/μl range; occasionally the total numbers are decreased and rarely a very high count is observed. The lymphocytes frequently show abnormal features, including a generalized pleomorphism of the cells which tend to be larger than normal. The nuclei may show primitive features having finely stippled chromatin and prominent nucleoli. The nucleus may be reniform or lobulated and this feature has led to some observers classifying the cells as monocytes. The cytoplasm is more abundant than in the usual lymphocyte; it may be a deeper blue and frequently contains many azurophil granules and vacuoles. Usually a few typical plasma cells are also present and there is often an increase in the number of monocytes. Anaemia is not usual, but may be present due to a pre-existing cause, and occasionally is due to haemolysis. The platelet count is usually normal but thrombocytopenia causing purpura or mucosal haemorrhage is occasionally found.

Serum antibodies

The serum usually contains heterophil antibodies which will agglutinate sheep red cells. Unfortunately, this Paul–Bunnell heterophil antibody test is not always positive or may only become positive in the convalescent stage of the disease. If negative in the acute stages the test should be repeated at a later date.

The sera of some normal individuals and that of patients immune to horse serum may contain antibodies which agglutinate sheep red cells. These can be differentiated by a differential absorption test. Aliquots of positive sera are treated with extracts of guinea-pig kidney and ox erythrocytes and then tested for their ability to agglutinate sheep red cells. The antibody of infectious mononucleosis is not absorbed by guinea-pig kidney but is by ox cells. A titre of 1 in 20 after absorption of the sera with guinea-pig kidney in suspension is strongly indicative and a 1 in 80 titre diagnostic of infectious mononucleosis. 'Normal' antibody is absorbed by guinea-pig kidney, but not by ox cells; that found in horse serum sensitivity is absorbed by both. Antibodies to the EB virus are demonstrable in the majority of subjects with infectious mononucleosis. In general, antibody levels rise rapidly and it is usually not possible to demonstrate a rising antibody titre unless blood has been obtained before the infection. EB antibody testing is not performed routinely because it is technically difficult. This antibody and the heterophil antibody have been shown to be different.

Diagnosis

A typical clinical picture and the presence of typical cells in the blood or a positive heterophil antibody test establish the diagnosis.

The condition may be confused with other causes of sore throat and other virus infections, especially viral hepatitis. In some of these conditions a few atypical lymphocytes may be found but they are not usually present in the numbers found in infectious mononucleosis, nor is the heterophil antibody test positive. Occasionally it may be difficult to exclude acute leukaemia.

Treatment

The disease may take a very variable course. Some patients recover rapidly whereas others are incapacitated for months. There is no specific treatment; rarely, corticosteroids are needed for such complications as thrombocytopenia or haemolytic anaemia.

Infectious lymphocytosis

In infectious lymphocytosis up to 100,000 lymphocytes/μl may be found in the blood and the bone marrow may be moderately infiltrated with similar cells. Morphologically the cells are normal and the condition remits after a few weeks or months. Although the condition is uncommon, it is important because it may be confused with chronic lymphocytic leukaemia. The natural history of the conditions differentiates the two. It is of low infectivity, but outbreaks may occur in closed communities.

Leukaemoid reaction

Occasionally in severe infections, drug reactions, malignant diseases and hepatic failure it is difficult to distinguish the blood picture of a reactive leucocytosis from that of leukaemia. The reactive leucocytosis differs in that it will remit when the causative disease is removed and by the fact that the shift to the left of the cells is usually less marked than in leukaemia. The leucocyte count is often higher in leukaemia than in a reactive leucocytosis.

A granulocytic leucocytosis can be differentiated from chronic granulocytic leukaemia by a cytochemical test for the presence of the enzyme, alkaline phosphatase, in the neutrophils (p. 131). It is practically absent from the neutrophils in chronic granulocytic leukaemia but large amounts are present in a reactive leucocytosis.

Infectious mononucleosis is sometimes confused with acute leukaemia. The presence of a positive heterophil antibody test confirms a diagnosis of infectious mononucleosis. Anaemia and thrombocytopenia, which may be present occasionally in infectious mononucleosis, are much commoner in cases of acute leukaemia.

Leucopenia

In leucopenia the total leucocyte count is reduced below 4,000/μl. The condition is usually due to decreased neutrophils, but is occasionally due to a decrease in the lymphocytes.

Neutropenia and agranulocytosis

Neutropenia and agranulocytosis may occur as part of a generalized depression of haemopoiesis (hypoplastic pancytopenia or aplastic anaemia) or the granulocytes may be selectively depressed. When the condition is severe (usually with less than 500 neutrophils/μl) the term agranulocytosis is used. Less severe forms (with neutrophil counts between 500 and 2,000/μl) are called neutropenia.

Both conditions are usually secondary to some other disorder, but occasionally occur without any obvious cause, in which case they are termed idiopathic. Overwhelming infections and those in which there is a lymphocytosis or monocytosis are sometimes associated with a neutropenia. Another common cause is bone marrow damage due to irradiation, toxic drugs (phenylbutazone, chloramphenicol, anti-epileptic drugs, antithyroid drugs and cytotoxic drugs), or disturbances due to primary or secondary malignant disorders. Neutropenia may also occur following blood transfusion, in which case it is thought that leucocyte antibodies are responsible. Active systemic lupus erythematosus is also frequently associated with leucopenia due to leucocyte antibodies. The neutrophil numbers are depressed and there is a shift to the right in folate and cobalamin deficiency, and hypersplenism is usually associated with neutropenia. A further condition, called cyclic neutropenia, is also recognized in which the neutrophils periodically disappear from the blood. This condition is thought to be inherited, both autosomal dominant and recessive nodes of transmission being found.

The clinical features depend upon the severity of the neutropenia and its cause. In agranulocytosis the condition is usually acute and severe. Infections, usually of the mouth or throat, are common and ulceration may be present. Fever, pneumonia and septicaemia may follow and the condition is frequently fatal. In the less severe and in chronic forms, infections for which there are no obvious causes are frequent. The spleen may be palpable and the lymph nodes draining the area of infection are often enlarged. The condition may remit either spontaneously or following the removal of the cause, or it may become more severe leading to septicaemia.

In patients who are receiving cytotoxic chemotherapy, the bone marrow granulocyte reserves may be tested by injecting bacterial endotoxin or, preferably, by using the steroid metabolite, etiocholanolone. In the presence of impaired reserves, an increment in the baseline white cell count of less than 2,600/μl is found.

Eosinopenia

Eosinophil counts of less than 100/μl may occur in hyperadrenalcorticoidism.

Basopenia

Basophil counts of less than 20/μl occur in allergic reactions and stress reaction. A special counting technique is required.

Lymphopenia

Lymphocyte counts of less than 1,000 cells/μl may be found in severe depressions of the leucopoietic tissues; for example, following treatment with radiation or cytotoxic drugs. It also may be found following the use of corticotrophin or steroid hormones and in severe congestive cardiac failure. Advanced Hodgkin's disease is also associated with lymphopenia.

Functional defects of neutrophils

In recent years, defects in the ability of neutrophils to phagocytose and kill bacteria have been described. These disorders may be congenital or acquired. Because of the imprecision with which neutrophil function can be assessed, their classification is not yet clear-cut.

Fatal chronic granulomatous disease of childhood is a rare, X-linked recessive entity characterized by recurrent systemic bacterial infections, skin infections varying from furuncles to chronic granulomatous infections with prominent accumulations of tissue histiocytes microscopically. There is decreased intracellular killing of common bacteria by both neutrophils and monocytes. More rarely, related congenital neutrophil defects are seen in girls, with an apparently sporadic occurrence and a clinical picture of recurrent infections without granuloma formation.

Acquired neutrophil dysfunction has been described in alcoholic intoxication and diabetic ketoacidosis.

Further reading

BRAUNSTEINER, H. and ZUCKER-FRANKLIN, D. (1962). *The Physiology and Pathology of Leukocytes.* Grune and Stratton, New York.

CARTER, R. L. and PENMAN, H. G. (1969). *Infectious Mononucleosis.* Blackwell Scientific, Oxford.

CRONKITE, E. P. and VINCENT, P. C. (1969). Granulocytopoiesis. *Ser. Haematol.* **2**, 3–43.

WINDHORST, D. B. (1970). Functional defects of neutrophils. *Advanc. intern. Med.* **16**, 329–49.

9 The leukaemias and paraproteinaemias

THE LEUKAEMIAS

General aspects

The leukaemias, lymphomas and allied disorders are characterized by an abnormal proliferation of the reticular and haemopoietic tissues. They are generally considered to be neoplasms and three overlapping groups may be distinguished. In the first a localized tumour is found, in the second the condition is generalized throughout the reticular tissue and in the third abnormal cells are also found in the blood. Those that involve the leucopoietic tissues are divided into the leukaemias, in which the blood usually contains abnormal cells, and the lymphomas (Chapter 10), in which the blood spread is less common. The distinction is convenient in that the leukaemias are usually diagnosed from blood and bone marrow examination and the lymphomas by lymph node or other biopsies. Amongst the related disorders are the myelomas (p. 134), the erythraemias (p. 104), idiopathic thrombocythaemia (p. 155) and myelofibrosis (p. 107).

Definition of leukaemia

The leukaemias are a group of disorders of uncertain aetiology characterized by an abnormal proliferation of the leucopoietic tissues of the body. They are almost invariably fatal although temporary remissions may occur.

The name leukaemia was given to the condition by Virchow because of the white appearance of the blood due to increased numbers of circulating white cells. Leucocythaemia is a better term but the name leukaemia is firmly established and is used to include not only cases in which there is a high concentration of leucocytes in the blood, the *leukaemic leukaemias*, but also those in which the numbers are not increased. If the total leucocyte count is normal or reduced but abnormal cells can be recognized in the blood then the term *subleukaemic* leukaemia is used. If, as occurs rarely, no abnormal cells are present in the blood then the condition is called *aleukaemic leukaemia*. To avoid this somewhat awkward nomenclature some prefer the term *leukosis* to leukaemia; this they qualify as leukaemic, subleukaemic or aleukaemic.

The nature and pathogenesis of leukaemia

Because of their proliferative and fatal features the leukaemias are accepted as malignant neoplasms. Superficial differences from other neoplasms include their possible multicentric origin and the occurrence of remissions. For these and other reasons, some consider that the neoplastic nature of these disorders is not established; however, most agree with the International Statistical Classification of Diseases which places the leukaemias among the malignant neoplasms of the lymphatic and haemopoietic tissues. The mechanisms by which normal leucocytes undergo the change which leads to their proliferation without normal maturation are unknown. The most plausible suggestion is that of a somatic mutation leading to an abnormal cell strain within the body, and the evidence certainly suggests that cellular rather than extracellular factors are the more important. Probably several different agents (or a combination), possibly through a multistep process, lead to an irreversible malignant transformation. The disorder of the regulation of leucocytes as between the tissue and the blood which occurs in cases of leukaemia has not yet been fully explained.

Incidence

The incidence of leukaemia, as reflected in the death rate, has been rising in Britain and some other countries during the last three decades and is now about 50 per 100,000 of the population. Part of the increase is attributed to better diagnosis and reporting but it is generally accepted that a real increase has occurred. This is especially so in the acute leukaemias of the older age groups. The high incidence in children, compared with other diseases, has also apparently increased but much of this may be due to the increased facilities for diagnosis which have been developed during the last 25 years. The incidence varies in different races and is generally higher in the more developed countries. The age and sex incidence of each variety of leukaemia are given in the appropriate section below.

Classification

The leukaemias are best classified clinically into acute and chronic and cytologically according to the predominant cell type. In the absence of treatment patients with acute leukaemia generally die within 3 months of diagnosis and the main cell involved in the process is usually a primitive cell; that is, a myeloblast, lymphoblast or a monocyte precursor. Patients with chronic leukaemia usually live for 1 or more years after the onset of the disease. The cells appear more mature, being mainly myelocytes or lymphocytes. Monocytic leukaemias are usually acute even when the cells appear to be mainly of a mature type. Some haematologists recognize a subacute type in which the untreated survival time is between 6 and 12 months or so.

The leukaemias may also be classified according to the tissue involved as myeloid or lymphoid, and the acute forms into childhood and adult types.

Aetiology

The cause of most cases of leukaemia is not known. There are probably many different factors of importance and they may differ for each type of leukaemia. However, at present it is simpler to consider all types together. A small proportion of leukaemias can definitely be ascribed to radiation; other possible causes are viruses, drugs and chemicals and genetic factors.

Radiation

Exposure to irradiation is a potent cause of leukaemia in animals and there is definite evidence that it can cause leukaemia in man. Analysis of leukaemias appearing in three groups—those exposed to radiation in their work, those who survived the atomic bomb explosions in Japan and patients exposed to therapeutic and diagnostic radiation—shows an incidence greater than expected.

Many of the pioneer workers in the use of radiation for medical purposes took inadequate precautions against excessive exposure. Case reports of leukaemia and other neoplasms in radiologists and their assistants suggest that there was an association between exposure and the disease. A survey of obituary notices of American doctors showed that physicians as a whole had a death rate from leukaemia two times, and radiologists eight times, that expected. Some of this increase may be attributed to increased facilities for the diagnosis of diseases in doctors but it is likely that, at least in the radiologists, it was occupational. British radiologists have not had this increased incidence of leukaemia, possibly because they have taken greater precautions against accidental exposure.

The survivors of the 1945 atomic explosions over Nagasaki and Hiroshima had an incidence of leukaemia greatly in excess of the average for Japan. Those within 1,000 metres of the explosion had a greatly increased incidence. A moderate increase occurred in those between 1,000 and 2,500 metres away and only a slight increase in those more than 2,500 metres from the explosion.

Patients exposed to therapeutic irradiation occasionally develop leukaemia and it is suggested that there is a direct connection between the treatment and the development of leukaemia. The patients include those treated with x-rays for non-malignant conditions such as skin lesions, enlargement of the thymus and ankylosing spondylitis and by radioactive iodine for the treatment of thyrotoxicosis. Statistical evidence that the association might be real was provided by a British Medical Research Council investigation into patients with ankylosing spondylitis treated with radiation. An incidence of leukaemia ten times greater than expected by chance was found but the possibility of an association between the disease, as opposed to the treatment and the leukaemia, was not excluded. The fact that the incidence was roughly correlated with the dosage of radiation received suggested a direct relationship between the two. A point not settled by this investigation and which is actively disputed is the possibility of a threshold dosage of radiation below which x-rays are not leukaemogenic. Since it is not possible to be certain that low dosage radiation is safe, it is wise to consider all ionizing radiation as potentially leukaemogenic. The increased risk of developing leukaemia following low doses, if real, must, however, be very small.

There is some evidence that the low dosages received in diagnostic radiation are leukaemogenic but this is not accepted by all. Some writers have found that children who have received total body radiation *in utero* during their mother's pregnancy are more likely to develop leukaemia than those who have not been irradiated, but the increased incidence is small and has not been confirmed in all series. Nevertheless, unnecessary exposure to radiation should be avoided, especially in pregnancy and during childhood.

Virus

Viruses are known to cause leukaemia in some animals and there is indirect evidence that they may be leukaemogenic for man. It has been known for many years that fowl leukaemias are due to a virus; in the last decade several mouse leukaemias, some of which resemble human leukaemias fairly closely, have been shown to be viral. However, the mouse leukaemia viruses do not spread like the usual infective agents, being transmitted only from parent to offspring through the gametes or experimentally by injection in fetuses or newborn mice. There is no direct evidence that human leukaemia is due to a virus and the infusion of leukaemic blood into humans has not resulted in any leukaemia developing in the recipients. However, in several studies virus-like particles have been found in leukaemic cells and plasma. Some viruses have also been isolated from leukaemic material but it is possible that they are 'passengers' rather than 'drivers'. Burkitt's lymphoma, a disease with localized malignant lymphoblastic tumours which resembles acute leukaemia, has several features suggesting that it might be of viral origin and a virus has been isolated from tumour material.

Another suggestion of an infective cause of leukaemia comes from the occurrence of leukaemia in clusters, where several cases occur in the same neighbourhood and at about the same time.

At present more active research into this question is going on and the next few years may allow a definite answer to be given to the question of viral leukaemogenesis.

Drugs and chemicals

Leukaemia has been reported as occurring after exposure to agents known to depress the bone marrow. Benzol, used in various industrial processes, is generally considered to be leukaemogenic. The evidence in the case of drugs, such as phenylbutazone, is inconclusive and the risk, if any, of developing leukaemia after their use is small.

Genetic factors

A genetic factor in leukaemia is suggested by reports of several cases of leukaemia in the same family and by the fact that animals can be inbred to produce high leukaemia strains.

Environmental factors are not, however, excluded and, in the animals at least, transfer of a virus by the gametes may be responsible for the findings.

Patients with Down's syndrome (trisomy 21) have an increased liability to develop leukaemia; this appears to be associated with the extra chromosome and in this sense is genetic.

Other possible aetiological factors

That leukaemia may be a deficiency disease is supported by an analogy with pernicious anaemia. Prior to the discovery of 'liver treatment', patients with this disorder showed many features resembling leukaemia. There was a progressive course ending in death and hyperplasia of erythroid cells in the bone marrow. No maturation factor has been found, however, and there is much evidence that the defect in leukaemia lies in the cell itself rather than in its environment.

Another theory is that leukaemia is due to a failure of elimination of mature cells by the lungs or other tissues, and yet another is that it represents the response of the body to some infecting micro-organisms.

ACUTE LEUKAEMIAS

The acute leukaemias can be divided according to the age of the patient into childhood and adult types, and according to the cell type involved into haemocytoblastic, lymphoblastic, myeloblastic and monoblastic or monocytic.

Childhood acute leukaemia

Acute leukaemias in children are differentiated from those found in adults by their clinical features and by their response to therapy. Of those with acute leukaemia, 90% will respond to treatment, whereas only about 50% of adults obtain a reasonable remission even with the most intensive treatment.

Classification and incidence

The majority of childhood leukaemias are lymphoblastic (labelled by some as 'haemocytoblastic' or 'stem cell' leukaemias); myeloblastic leukaemias occur not occasionally and monocytic cases are rare.

Congenital leukaemia is rare; incidence in childhood peaks in the age group 3–6 years, and has been rising in recent years. Much of this is probably secondary to increased facilities for diagnosis and the reduced mortality of childhood infections which followed the introduction of antibiotics. The incidence and death rate is about 0·5 per 100,000 in most Western countries.

Clinical features

The onset of the disease is usually acute. Presenting symptoms and signs include fever, bone pains, pallor, petechiae and bruising, lymphadenopathy, splenomegaly, signs of infection in the throat and elsewhere. In the absence of a remission, death follows within a few weeks due to haemorrhage, infection or profound anaemia. Spontaneous, or treatment-induced, remissions may occur and last for several months. Further remissions can sometimes be obtained, in which case the patient may survive for a year or more. Neurological complications may develop in treated patients who are otherwise well; these are due to leukaemic cells proliferating within the meninges where they are not affected by treatment and intrathecal therapy is needed.

Further complications include hyperuricaemia and renal failure. Death is usually due to infection, haemorrhage or profound anaemia.

Laboratory findings

Blood examination typically reveals normochromic normocytic anaemia and thrombocytopenia. The total leucocyte count may be raised, normal or lowered. Examination of the blood smears shows the presence of leukaemic lymphoblasts or, less commonly, myeloblasts. Rarely, no abnormal cells are seen in the peripheral blood; in such aleukaemic leukaemias the diagnosis is made on the bone marrow findings. The erythrocyte sedimentation rate is usually high.

The *bone marrow* is infiltrated with and often completely replaced by leukaemic blast cells. The other cells of the granulocytic, erythrocytic and megakaryocytic cell series are correspondingly depressed.

Diagnosis

The diagnosis, which may be suspected on clinical grounds, is confirmed by blood and bone marrow examinations. The differentiation into cell types is based on the morphology of the cells and their cytochemical reactions (see below, under 'Adult acute leukaemias'). Differentiation from infectious mononucleosis is sometimes difficult. Both anaemia and thrombocytopenia are commoner in leukaemia; the leucocytes in infectious mononucleosis do not usually show as markedly primitive features as those in an acute leukaemia and they are more pleomorphic. A positive Paul–Bunnell test is of value in confirming a diagnosis of infectious mononucleosis but unfortunately it is not always present, especially in the acute stage when confusion between the two diseases may occur.

In certain conditions, such as infections, drug reactions, malignant disease and hepatic failure, a leukaemoid reaction develops in the blood (p. 118).

Whilst granulocytic leukaemoid reactions are more usual, lymphocytic reactions can develop and cause diagnostic difficulty.

Treatment and course

The aim of treatment is to induce a remission in the disease because survival is very short without this. Treatment with cytotoxic drugs may accentuate complications due to the disease, especially the bleeding of thrombocytopenia and infections from neutropenia. Thus adequate facilities for supportive management are required. These include facilities for nursing the patient in a sterile environment, good microbiological laboratory facilities and the availability of platelet transfusions. Corticosteroids may be used for thrombocytopenic haemorrhage.

The previous chemotherapeutic approach in acute leukaemia was to give one drug continuously until resistance developed and then change to another. This approach was supplanted by cyclical therapy and combination therapy.

The drugs of choice for *remission induction* in acute leukaemia are vincristine 1·4 mg/m^2 I.V. weekly and prednisone 40 mg/m^2 daily by mouth. With this combination a complete remission may be expected in 90% of patients. A complete remission is defined as a return to good health, the absence of physical abnormalities, normality of the blood and bone marrow and the absence of leukaemic infiltration in the nervous system or other organs.

If remission is not achieved with vincristine and prednisone, then the combination of the antipyrimidine, cytosine arabinoside and the antibiotic daunorubicin should be used. The enzyme, L-asparaginase is also used by some. This drug should not be used alone because resistance rapidly develops.

When complete remission is obtained, a period of *cytoreduction therapy* is undertaken with the antipurine, 6-mercaptopurine, and the folate antagonist, methotrexate. Some also use L-asparaginase at this time. There is considerable variation in the intensity of therapy regimens in various centres at this particular stage. Frequently, because of the proclivity for meningeal leukaemia to develop in remission, prophylactic intrathecal methotrexate, with or without irradiation to the neuraxis, is given. Central nervous system involvement develops because of the failure of most anti-leukaemic drugs to cross the blood–brain barrier.

Finally, maintenance therapy is given, usually methotrexate twice weekly and mercaptopurine daily and, in some centres, repeated courses of combination chemotherapy ('reinduction therapy'). Immunotherapy is given by some at this stage but its value has yet to be proved and it is only effective in patients with minimal amounts of leukaemic tissue. Non-specific therapy with BCG and specific therapy with killed autologous lymphoblasts are the usual forms of immunotherapy.

Median survival with these regimens is now 3 years or more, and some patients survive much longer. Relapse and death from infection or haemorrhage ultimately occur, although a few cases of apparent cures are now being reported.

Adult acute leukaemias

Adult acute leukaemia may present as a primary disorder or follow an aplastic anaemia or chronic granulocytic leukaemia.

Classification and incidence

The majority are myeloblastic or monocytic; lymphoblastic types are uncommon. If cells of both the myeloblastic and monocytic cell series are present the condition is called myelomonocytic leukaemia. This mixed or Naegeli form may be distinguished from the pure monocytic or Schilling form. The incidence of adult acute leukaemia is greater in the older age group and has risen appreciably over the last decade so that it is now the commonest form of leukaemia in Western countries. The incidence rises from about 0·25 per 100,000 in middle age to 1 per 100,000 in the elderly.

Clinical features

The onset may be gradual with generalized ill health, lassitude, anorexia, dyspnoea and pallor over several weeks or months. Infections and bruising are common; lymphadenopathy or haemorrhage may be the presenting symptom. Splenomegaly is not usually marked; if a large hard spleen is felt, a previous chronic granulocytic leukaemia may have been present. Hypertrophy of the gums and bleeding in the mouth are common early symptoms, especially in monocytic leukaemia. Retinal haemorrhages may cause disturbances of vision.

In general it is true to say that the manifestations are due first to depression of normal red cells, granulocytes and platelets, and second to the toxaemia of the disease itself.

A few cases develop localized greenish tumour masses called chloromas which produce local pressure effects, such as paraplegia if they occur in the epidural space of the spinal canal.

Laboratory findings

A normochromic normocytic anaemia is almost always present. Leukaemic blast cells are present in the peripheral blood, usually in increased numbers; less commonly there is a subleukaemic picture. The platelets are reduced in numbers and sometimes absent. The bone marrow is infiltrated with leukaemic blast cells which form at least 30% and sometimes over 95% of the cells present.

The morphological type of the leukaemic cells may be assessed from their appearance in the stained films, from the presence of other leucocytes in the smear, from cytochemical stains and other special tests. Leukaemic myeloblasts vary in diameter from 10 to 20 μm, have large finely reticulated nuclei, contain 2–5 nucleoli and an intensely blue cytoplasm. The nucleus is sometimes folded or lobulated. The cytoplasm does not usually contain inclusions but sometimes azurophil needle-like crystals (Auer bodies) and granules are present. These cells merge into leukaemic promyelocytes which contain many azurophil granules and allow the leukaemia to be classified as myeloblastic. Generally there is an absence of myelocytes and metamyelocytes (the hiatus leukaemicus); occasional segmented neutrophils are usually present and may show nuclear abnormalities.

Leukaemic myeloblasts and promyelocytes containing azurophil granules are usually peroxidase and sudan-black positive. This helps to distinguish them from leukaemic lymphoblasts; unfortunately, very 'primitive' myeloblasts may be negative.

Leukaemic lymphoblasts are similar to leukaemic myeloblasts but usually contain less cytoplasm, which may be irregular. The nuclear pattern is perhaps coarser and typically contains only one or two nucleoli. The cytoplasm may be vacuolated but granules are rare and Auer bodies are not seen. The blast cells are peroxidase negative and contain only a few fine sudan-black-positive granules. The cells often contain coarse PAS-positive granules in the cytoplasm; these are not seen in myeloblasts.

In monoblastic leukaemia the predominant cell is usually a leukaemic promonocyte; leukaemic monoblasts are less common and resemble leukaemic myeloblasts. The leukaemic promonocytes are large cells, 15–25 μm in diameter, with folded or indented nuclei. The chromatin network is somewhat coarser than in blast cells and consists of long strands rather than dots or lumps. Nucleoli are faint or absent. The cytoplasm is abundant, moderately basophilic, opaque and often has an irregular outline. Azurophil granules are usually present and occasionally Auer bodies are seen. Leukaemic monocytes which resemble normal monocytes are usually present in increased numbers.

The peroxidase and PAS reaction are negative or slightly positive. In the sudan-black reaction the cells contain diffusely scattered small black granules.

The segmented neutrophils are said to have a weak alkaline phosphatase reaction but this is not invariable.

In myelomonocytic (Naegeli) leukaemias, myelocytic and monocytic cells are present together.

Diagnosis

The diagnosis is usually suspected clinically and confirmed upon examination of the peripheral blood and bone marrow. Differentiation from infectious mononucleosis and leukaemoid reactions may cause difficulty (p. 118).

Treatment and course

As with childhood leukaemia, the aim is to induce a remission. However, this is much more difficult to achieve in acute myeloblastic leukaemia and, once achieved, remissions are usually short-lived.

An attempt to achieve a remission is usually made with a combination of cytosine arabinoside and daunorubicin. About half will have a complete remission with this regimen; usually, however, it will be at the expense of a period of severe bone marrow hypoplasia. Facilities for sterile nursing and frequent swabs of body orifices for pathogenic organisms are required. Septicaemia occurs frequently, often with unusual organisms, and intensive antibacterial chemotherapy will be required. Thrombocytopenic haemorrhage is often a problem and is treated with corticosteroids and platelet transfusions.

Survival when a remission is obtained is usually 6–12 months, but if no remission is achieved, survival is mostly only a period of 3 months or less.

Maintenance therapy is with twice weekly methotrexate and with daily mercaptopurine in a dose such as to cause mild but tolerable bone marrow suppression.

Once relapse occurs, cytosine arabinoside and daunorubicin are tried again, but usually with limited success and most patients rapidly die of infection or haemorrhage.

CHRONIC LEUKAEMIAS

Chronic granulocytic leukaemia

A disease of middle age and old age, chronic granulocytic leukaemia has a peak incidence in the fifties. It is less common than acute leukaemia, having an incidence of about 1 per 100,000. The sex ratio is equal.

Clinical features

The onset of the disease is insidious and careful questioning may reveal that symptoms have been present for many months before the diagnosis is made. Vague ill health is usually common and either that or pain or enlargement of the spleen may be the reason for seeking medical advice. Loss of weight, fever and symptoms of anaemia are other modes of presentation. Haemorrhage is sometimes the presenting feature.

Laboratory findings

A moderate normochromic normocytic anaemia is usually found; this generally becomes more severe during the course of the disease but usually remits during successful treatment.

The leucocyte count is usually raised to between 50,000 and 350,000 cells/μl. Many of the cells are leukaemic myelocytes and metamyelocytes. A few leukaemic myeloblasts and promyelocytes are also present; if they form more than 10%, it may indicate that an 'acute' transformation is occurring. About 50% of the cells are usually segmented granulocytes. In the rarer neutrophilic leukaemia, over 90% of the leucocytes are neutrophil metamyelocytes and segmented cells. The proportion of both basophils and eosinophils to neutrophils is often considerably greater than normal.

The platelet count is usually raised in the early stages, being in the region of 500,000-1,000,000/μl; in the late stages there may be thrombocytopenia.

The serum uric acid may be grossly raised due to the increased nucleoprotein turnover, as in the other leukaemias.

The enzyme, alkaline phosphatase, usually present in mature neutrophils can be demonstrated histochemically and its activity expressed numerically as a score. One hundred mature neutrophils are examined and given a score of 0 to 4 depending on the intensity of the staining reaction. Of the possible score of 0 to 400, most blood rates 15 to 100. The activity in chronic granulocytic leukaemia is decreased and may be 0. This is possibly due to cytoplasmic immaturity in CGL neutrophils. With a remission of the disease, the score rises; this is also seen in acute blast cell transformation. This test is useful in differentiating chronic granulocytic leukaemia from other myeloproliferative syndromes where neutrophil alkaline phosphatase activity will be found to be normal or characteristically high.

When chromosome preparations are made from the bone marrow or blood, a small abnormal chromosome called the Philadelphia (Ph^1) chromosome is found, so called because of the city where it was first described. The Ph^1 chromosome replaces one of the normal G group chromosomes, probably number 21, with the deletion of part of one of the long arms. It is found in all typical cases of chronic granulocytic leukaemia, and the abnormality does not disappear following a successful course of therapy of the disease. Since the abnormality is also present in megakaryoblasts and erythroblasts, these cells must be derived from a common precursor and the disease is one of the myeloid tissues rather than the granulocytic series alone.

Diagnosis

A diagnosis which may be suspected clinically from the history and gross splenomegaly is usually confirmed by the blood findings. Leukaemoid reaction with a marked neutrophil leucocytosis sometimes mimics leukaemia. The presence of more primitive cells is generally less marked in a leukaemoid reaction and the segmenting granulocytes are strongly positive when stained for alkaline phosphatase activity. Chromosomal preparations of the bone marrow (or of the blood, in relapse) will reveal the presence of the Ph^1 chromosome.

Treatment

Blood transfusions, antimicrobial chemotherapy and other symptomatic treatments are given as required.

Busulphan, an oral alkylating agent which acts more particularly against granulocytic cells, is the specific drug of choice. It is given in an initial daily dosage of 0·06 mg/kg body weight (to a maximum dose of 4 mg). The patient is seen every week or two, depending on the rate of fall of the white cell count, and treatment is suspended when the total white cell count reaches 20,000–15,000/μl. Continuation of the drug beyond this point can result in irreversible bone marrow depression.

With successful therapy, clinical improvement is marked, the anaemia ameliorated and the spleen regresses considerably and may become impalpable. Dibromomannitol, hydroxyurea, Colcemid and mercaptopurine are useful but less effective agents.

The alternative to drug therapy is radiation, which is somewhat less effective; this may be given as splenic irradiation or as radioactive phosphorus by mouth or intravenously.

Treatment induces a clinical remission in the vast majority of cases but the disease usually relapses after several months. If one of the therapies is ineffective the other may be tried and is often of benefit since there is no cross-resistance.

Some advise maintenance therapy with busulphan, titrating the daily dose against the leucocyte count, such as to maintain a total leucocyte count of between 10,000 and 20,000/μl. There is no evidence that ultimate survival is different whether continuous or intermittent therapy is given.

Course

The disease usually runs a course of 1–5 years. Treatment makes life more comfortable for the patients but does not have a great effect on the final outcome. In the majority of cases, acute leukaemia develops terminally. Treatment of the acute blast cell transformation is the same as for adult acute myeloblastic leukaemia, but the response is very poor and few patients achieve a remission. Death is usually due to anaemia, haemorrhage of infection.

Chronic lymphocytic leukaemia

Incidence

Chronic lymphocytic leukaemia is usually a disease of old age, with an increase in incidence from about 0·25 per 100,000 in the fifties to 1 per 100,000 in the seventies. It is less common than acute leukaemia and slightly more common than chronic granulocytic leukaemia. There is a male to female ratio of about 2:1.

Clinical features

In some subjects the disease may run a benign course without appreciable symptoms, being detected incidentally. Some of these patients die of other causes and the leukaemia appears to be merely incidental. In others, however, the disorder is more malignant, causing symptoms and death within a year or so. The presenting symptoms and signs are variable; they include general debility and symptoms of anaemia, enlargement of the lymph nodes and spleen, skin rashes, purpura and other haemorrhagic manifestations, recurrent infections and the effects of mediastinal or intra-abdominal lymphadenopathy.

Laboratory findings

A normochromic normocytic anaemia of moderate degree is usual. In the terminal stages the anaemia may be severe. An associated haemolytic anaemia is found in about 15% of cases; the blood findings then include a reticulocytosis and a positive Coombs' test (p. 66). In some patients there is a hypogammaglobulinaemia which is associated with a poor response to infection. In some cases, the serum may contain a macroglobulin; these patients form about 5% and must be differentiated from the related lympho-proliferative disorder, Waldenström's macroglobulinaemia.

The leucocyte count is generally raised to between 50,000 and 250,000/μl, but higher and lower values are sometimes seen. The majority of the cells are leukaemic lymphocytes, usually small and frequently indistinguishable from normal lymphocytes, especially in the more benign cases. Larger cell types with more abundant cytoplasm and many smear cells are sometimes seen; this is often associated with a more rapid clinical course. The platelets are normal or reduced in number; terminally there may be thrombo-cytopenia.

The bone marrow is usually infiltrated with lymphocytes which usually form at least 50% of the nucleated cells present. The other cells are proportionally decreased.

Diagnosis

The diagnosis may be suspected on clinical grounds but requires confirmation by blood and bone marrow examinations.

Treatment

Blood transfusions, antibacterial chemotherapy, immunoglobulin G and other symptomatic treatments are given as indicated. For asymptomatic patients no therapy is required. Corticosteroid therapy may cause lympholysis and is especially valuable if an autoimmune haemolytic anaemia is present. Chlorambucil, an oral alkylating agent, is effective in reducing the leucocyte count and lymph nodes in most cases. Cyclophosphamide or other alkylating agents may be used.

Radiotherapy is also effective; 'titrated' doses of total body irradiation or radioactive phosphorus in doses designed to reduce the leucocyte count to 10,000–20,000 are given. Radiotherapy may also be given to enlarged lymph nodes or spleen.

Splenectomy is occasionally of value if the spleen size is causing symptoms or if haemolysis does not respond to steroid therapy.

Course

The course of the disease varies tremendously from a rapidly fatal outcome in less than a year to a chronic course of over 15 years. Most patients, however, die within 5 years of diagnosis. Unlike chronic granulocytic leukaemia, a terminal acute phase is uncommon; death is usually due to infection, anaemia or haemorrhage.

THE PARAPROTEINAEMIAS

Introduction

Immunoglobulins are a group of γ-globulins produced by plasma cells and certain lymphocytes associated with antibody activity. They share four linked polypeptide chains in common, two heavy (H) and two light. There are two types of light chains, kappa (κ) and lambda (λ). The heavy chains are different for each immunoglobulin and result in the different immunoglobulins, called IgG, IgA, IgM, IgD and IgE. If a single clone of plasma cells proliferates and produces a single protein, a sharp spike or monoclonal peak ('M component') is found on electrophoresis of the serum proteins on paper or other media. This component will contain immunoglobulin determinants of a single type of heavy chain and of a single type of light chain, confirming its monoclonal nature. This is in contrast to the normal antibody response where a single protein contains a number of antigens and elicits a polyclonal immunoglobulin response, showing as a diffuse band on serum protein electrophoresis. The diseases due to a monoclonal proliferation are called *monoclonal gammopathies* and the protein is called a paraprotein. The cells producing these discrete proteins are sometimes called *immunocytes* and thus a monoclonal proliferation may be said to be due to an immunocytoma.

If the plasma cell clone producing this protein behaves in a malignant fashion, then the disease is called multiple myeloma.

Benign monoclonal gammopathy

On occasion, especially in population surveys, a monoclonal protein is discovered by chance and it may be questioned whether this is a benign condition or whether it represents early myelomatosis. Waldenström has described an entity, which he termed *benign essential hyperglobulinaemia,* when a paraprotein is found which persists unchanged for many years without evidence of disease. The characteristics of this group of patients are (1) serum paraprotein level of less than 1 g/100 ml, (2) persistence but not increase in the paraprotein level when followed over a period of 5 years or more, (3) no quantitative decrease in the other normal immunoglobulin levels, (4) the absence of immunoglobulin fragments such as free light chains (Bence–Jones protein) in the serum or urine, and (5) the absence of plasma cells or lymphoid cells infiltrating the bone marrow.

Multiple myeloma

The term myeloma was first applied to solitary tumours of the bone marrow, and multiple myelomatosis to the more common generalized involvement of the medullary bones. It was later found that these tumours were almost all composed of plasma cells and the term plasmacytoma was used. The term myeloma has, however, become established and is applied also to those plasmacytomas which may be found in reticular tissue other than the bone marrow and occasionally in other sites. Multiple myelomatosis likewise may involve tissues other than the bone marrow, either primarily or, more commonly, concomitantly with bone marrow involvement. The solitary myelomas can occasionally be treated successfully with surgery; some remain localized for some time but the majority spread and transform into multiple myelomas.

This condition is a malignant proliferation of the plasma cells throughout the bone marrow and other tissues associated with the production of immunoglobulins or immunoglobulin fragments found in the serum or urine. Some classify the condition according to the cytology of the abnormal plasma cells, most now according to the types of abnormal protein produced. The term plasma cell leukaemia is used if there are an appreciable number of neoplastic plasma cells in the peripheral blood.

The condition is uncommon but not rare, having an incidence of about 0·25 per 100,000. It occurs mainly in persons over 50 years of age, and there is a male to female ratio of 2:1. Nothing is known of the aetiology of the condition, which is classified as a malignant neoplasm.

Clinical features

Many of the symptoms and signs are due to the suppression of normal bone marrow function by the abnormal cells and to the production of the abnormal protein. They include bone pain, pathological fractures and progressive anaemia. Characteristic x-ray changes may be seen in the bones. These are osteolytic lesions without any surrounding reactive osteosclerosis, but diffuse osteoporosis also occurs. Recurrent infections due to deficiencies of normal immunoglobulins and sometimes leucopenia are often a problem. Some patients present with a bleeding diathesis; this may be due to thrombocytopenia or to interference with platelet function by the abnormal protein. On occasion, the paraprotein may interfere with coagulation factor function—most often by the inhibition of the bonding of fibrin monomers. It has been shown that the paraprotein binds to fibrinogen and is present in the resultant abnormal fibrin clot.

Renal failure is common and this is most often due to deposition of Bence-Jones protein in the renal tubules. Other causes are the deposition of amyloid in association with the myeloma, hypercalcaemic nephropathy or uric acid nephropathy. Infection such as pyelonephritis may also develop. The deposition of amyloid also causes features such as cardiomyopathy, macroglossia or peripheral neuropathy as an infrequent problem. The origin of amyloid has been a vexing and fascinating problem. Recent evidence suggests that amyloid fibrils are derived from variable regions of light chain fragments. This is more prone to occur with λ light chains.

Laboratory findings

Laboratory examination usually reveals a moderate to severe anaemia which is usually normochromic and normocytic but which may be macrocytic. The leucocytes are usually normal but in some cases leukaemic plasma cells are seen. The thrombocytes are normal or reduced in numbers. The erythrocyte sedimentation rate and plasma viscosity are usually raised (unless the myeloma is producing light chains only) and an abnormal protein can be demonstrated by serum electrophoresis in the β- or γ-globulin region. Sedimentation studies show that these proteins usually have a Svedberg constant of about 7, and immunologically they are IgA,

IgG or, less often, IgD. Rarely, myelomatosis is associated with a macroglobulin with a Svedberg constant of 7 (instead of 19) which is immunologically related to IgM. The plasma calcium level is often high. In up to 80% of cases the concentrated urine contains excess protein which has a mobility in the β or γ range but a smaller molecular weight than in the serum. Often this protein has the property of precipitating on warming to 50–70°C and redissolving at 90–100°C (Bence–Jones protein). It is formed of part of the molecules (light chains) of the abnormal protein produced by the plasma cells; it can be demonstrated in small amounts in the serum but, because of its low molecular weight, it is rapidly excreted.

Myeloma due to IgG forms about half of all cases of myeloma. There is an associated depression of normal immunoglobulins and consequently a greater predisposition to infection. The level of paraprotein is usually higher than the other types although the growth rate is slower. About one-quarter of the cases are IgA myeloma and have more frequent hypercalcaemia. Amyloidosis and increased light chain urinary excretion are frequent.

The finding of light chains or other fragments with the immunoglobulin indicates 'biochemical dedifferentiation' of the immunocytoma and that there is imbalance in heavy and light chain synthesis. This usually is associated with a more aggressive clinical course of the disease. In about one-fifth of the cases, light chains only are found in the serum and urine (Bence–Jones myeloma). This further biochemical dedifferentiation is expressed as a usually rapidly progressive disease with more bony destruction, hypercalcaemia, amyloidosis and renal failure. Myeloma due to IgD tends to behave like Bence–Jones myeloma, and many show extraosseous plasmacytomas. Rarely, an IgM paraprotein is associated with a classical clinical picture of myeloma and on occasion no paraprotein may be found at all. The occurrence of heavy chains as a paraprotein is associated with a lymphomatous clinical disease. Various incomplete molecular fragments are found rarely; these usually accompany an atypical clinical picture.

Bone marrow examination shows a partial to almost complete replacement of normal cells by abnormal plasma cells. They are usually pleomorphic, often have primitive nuclear features and abnormal cytoplasmic inclusions and giant cell formation is not uncommon.

Diagnosis

Diagnosis depends upon demonstrating the abnormal protein in the serum or urine and in the bone marrow appearances. Bony changes seen on x-ray may also be valuable. Differentiation from secondary hypergammaglobulinaemia due to liver disease, sarcoidosis, rheumatoid arthritis, disseminated lupus erythematosus and chronic infection depends upon the clinical history and nature of the protein. Differentiation from other causes of amyloid disease may also be required. Occasionally the condition is mistaken for chronic lymphocytic leukaemia since the abnormal plasma cells sometimes seen in the blood may have relatively scanty cytoplasm and may be confused with small lymphocytes.

Treatment and course

Radiotherapy is very valuable in alleviating bone pain or local pressure symptoms such as paraplegia. There is no evidence that ultimate survival is affected, however, and this is not unexpected since it is a systemic disease.

Of the cytotoxic drugs, only the alkylating agents phenylalanine mustard (melphalan; Alkeran, Sarolysin) and cyclophosphamide (Endoxana) have given favourable results, usually causing objective improvement in about 30% of patients and subjective improvement in a further percentage. Melphalan has been used more frequently but there is no evidence yet that it is superior to cyclophosphamide. The combination of melphalan and prednisone has been claimed to give superior results. This remains to be confirmed.

There is still no general agreement on the most effective dosage. The current principle of therapy is to use higher doses in intermittent courses. Melphalan is given in a dose of 0·1 mg/kg for 7–10 days, but dosage is dependent on marrow reserve. The drug is excreted in the urine and the dose must be reduced in the presence of renal failure. Cyclophosphamide may be given in full doses in the presence of renal insufficiency and, since it has the advantage of causing less platelet depression, it is preferred when pre-existent thrombocytopenia is a problem. The usual dose of cyclophosphamide is 200 mg I.V. daily for 10 days. Following bone marrow recovery, if maintenance therapy is to be given, then 50–100 mg cyclophosphamide daily is the usual dose, depending on marrow tolerance. Maintenance therapy with melphalan is usually 2 mg daily or every 2 days, again 'titrated' against the marrow reserve.

Complications such as hyperuricaemia may be controlled with allopurinol in a dose of approximately 300 mg. Hypercalcaemia is treated with corticosteroid therapy, usually prednisone 60–80 mg daily and a high fluid intake. Melphalan is also often efficacious in controlling hypercalcaemia. Not infrequently hypercalcaemia is resistant to these measures and intravenous or oral sodium phosphate may then be tried.

Bad prognostic features in myeloma include the presence of renal failure and heavy Bence–Jones proteinuria. A low serum albumin also connotes a poor prognosis.

Waldenström's macroglobulinaemia

Waldenström's macroglobulinaemia, a rarer condition, is allied to lymphosarcoma and to myeloma. It is a malignant lymphoreticular disorder associated with the production of high molecular weight macroglobulin having a Svedberg constant of 19 and immunologically belonging to the IgM group.

Clinical features

The onset of the illness is usually insidious with painless lymphadenopathy and splenomegaly, symptoms of easy bruising or other symptoms of a haemorrhagic diathesis. Frequently the patient presents with manifestations of serum hyperviscosity, including anorexia, lassitude, dizziness, haemorrhage, visual disturbances and disturbances of the conscious state. On examination the lymphadenopathy and splenomegaly are found; there may be purpuric haemorrhages, and the optic fundi may show distended retinal veins with haemorrhages and exudates. On occasion, retinal vein thrombosis occurs. These manifestations of hyperviscosity are made worse by cold weather.

Laboratory findings

Electrophoresis of serum proteins will reveal an abnormal discrete band which immunologically will be found to be IgM. The concentration is frequently up to 8 g/100 ml or more and its presence is usually associated with a gross increase in serum viscosity, accounting for the clinical features of hyperviscosity. Unlike myeloma, the non-involved immunoglobulins are usually not depressed.

Normochromic normocytic anaemia is usually found. This is also accompanied by an increase in plasma volume greater than would be expected for the degree of anaemia. The explanation for this is the oncotic effect of the IgM in increasing the entry of water into the vascular compartment. There may be moderate depression of white cells and platelets. Increased rouleaux formation and a high erythrocyte sedimentation rate are found.

Characteristically, bone marrow is difficult to aspirate and is found to be infiltrated with cells whose appearances are intermediate between plasma cells and lymphocytes. Sometimes the cells are indistinguishable from small lymphocytes. There is varying suppression of the normal cell lines.

Diagnosis

The clinical picture and laboratory findings are usually diagnostic. However, on occasion other lymphoproliferative disorders may be associated with the production of IgM paraprotein and a lymph node biopsy should be obtained if pathologically enlarged nodes are present. The histological appearances are of lymphocytic infiltration through the capsules, preservation of the sinus and medullary reticulin pattern, partial or complete absence of peripheral follicles, increase in most cell numbers and characteristic intranuclear inclusions found with the PAS stain.

Treatment and course

Basic treatment is directed at chemotherapeutic suppression of the IgM produced by the abnormal cells. Frequently the most pressing problem is that of the hyperviscosity syndrome. This can be controlled by regular plasmapheresis to reduce the plasma viscosity, blood being removed by phlebotomy and the plasma separated by either centrifugation or sedimentation of red cells, which are then infused back into the patient, the plasma being discarded. If preferred, an exchange transfusion of packed cells can be given during phlebotomy.

Chlorambucil or cyclophosphamide have been found to be the most effective cytotoxic drugs. The preferred mode of administration is on a prolonged, low dosage basis.

The disease may be variable in response. Some patients have a benign illness easily controlled with cytotoxic therapy. In others, regular plasmaphaeresis is needed to control hyperviscosity symptoms.

Further reading

BERNARD, J., JACQUILLAT, C. and WEIL, M. (1972). Treatment of the acute leukemias. *Semin. Hemat.* **9**, 181–91.

CLARKSON, B. D. and FRIED, J. (1971). Changing concepts of treatment in acute leukemia. *Med. Clin. N. Amer.* **55**, 561–600.

GALTON, D. A. G. (1969). Chemotherapy of chronic myelocytic leukemia. *Semin. Hemat.* **6**, 323–43.

SILVER, R. T. (1969). The treatment of chronic lymphocytic leukemia. *Semin. Hemat.* **6**, 344–56.

WALDENSTRÖM, J. (1968). Annotation. Treatment of multiple myeloma. *Brit. J. Haemat.* **15**, 217–20.

10 The lymphoproliferative disorders

General aspects

Introduction

Neoplastic changes in the lymphatic tissues give rise to a number of disorders which are conveniently collected together under the title of malignant lymphomas. They differ from the leukaemias in that the peripheral blood does not show any characteristic changes and the disorders may, at least at first, be localized to one site. The lymphomas resemble the leukaemias in that they are abnormal proliferations of the leucopoietic tissues; they are often fatal but on occasion they may be cured by radiotherapy. The incidence of the disorders is about 0·5 per 1,000 of the population in Britain; they are commoner than the leukaemias but less common than tumours such as carcinoma of the breast and bronchus. They may be classified on histological grounds into four groups—follicular lymphoma, reticulum cell sarcoma, lymphosarcoma and Hodgkin's disease. Each of these groups may be subdivided and intermediate types may also be found. The cause of these tumours is unknown but, at least for Burkitt's lymphoma, a viral aetiology seems likely. There is also some suggestion that there may be a genetic predisposition.

Clinical features

The clinical course is very variable. Some patients are little affected by their disease whereas in others it is rapidly fatal; a comparatively benign disorder may become rapidly malignant for no apparent reason. The patients usually present with enlargement of the lymph nodes, spleen or other lymphatic tissues. In the more generalized disorders constitutional disturbances including anorexia, weight loss, fever and symptoms of anaemia may be found.

Laboratory findings

The diagnosis and classification of these disorders depends upon histological examination of the affected tissues. The differentiation from reactive lymphatic hyperplasia of the lymphoid tissues is sometimes difficult and expert histological opinion is required. Blood examination usually shows no specific features but in some cases, especially in the later stages, the abnormal cells may be found in the peripheral blood. Anaemia and other changes due to infiltration of the bone marrow may also be found.

Treatment and course

The treatment depends upon the site and extent of the disease, its histological type and the general condition of the patient. Surgical removal of all the tumour tissue is possible in a very few cases. Radiotherapy is frequently given and is especially valuable for localized lesions. The type and dosage of radiation will depend upon the patient's clinical condition and the facilities available; it must be prescribed by a qualified radiotherapist and is available only in the larger hospitals. Chemotherapy may be preferred when the lesions are generalized or if radiotherapy is not available. It can be prescribed by all doctors but laboratory facilities must be available since all the agents used can cause depression of the bone marrow as well as other toxic side-effects. Results of treatment are better when given by doctors experienced in the use of such drugs and where feasible the patient should be referred to special centres for treatment.

The alkylating agents are the most useful group of drugs for these conditions. They cause their effects by alkylating two opposing guanine molecules on two strands of DNA, preventing the replication of DNA. Nitrogen mustard is still used by some doctors; it has to be given intravenously (0·4 mg/kg body weight in two divided doses is one regimen), diluted in saline with precautions against chemical phlebitis because it is a strong vesicant. Therapy is often complicated by nausea and vomiting. This can be partly controlled with the antiemetic drug, metoclopramide 10 mg I.V. beforehand. The major advantage of nitrogen mustard is its speed of action and it is used in emergency situations such as superior vena caval obstruction or spinal cord compression by the lymphomatous tissue. Chlorambucil (10 mg daily) is a suitable alternative which can be given orally; cyclophosphamide (200 mg daily), which can be given either intravenously or orally, is also effective. Both these drugs may cause alimentary upsets as well as marrow depression, and patients on cyclophosphamide may develop alopecia or haemorrhagic cystitis.

Corticosteroid drugs have a lymphocytolytic effect on the tumours in some cases.

Patients whose disease is resistant to the drugs already mentioned may be given one of the vinca alkaloids (vinblastine or vincristine); these occasionally produce a good result but have a number of undesirable side-effects. Vinblastine may cause neutropenia and whilst vincristine is far less myelotoxic, it is frequently associated with neurotoxicity to the peripheral and autonomic nervous system.

One of the synthetic methylhydrazines, procarbazine, has been found to be effective in Hodgkin's disease but not in the other lymphomas or in solid tumours. The more recent use of combinations of chemotherapeutic agents is discussed under the individual diseases.

Very frequently in these disorders, supportive management will be required. Anaemia due to bone marrow infiltration or depression from cytotoxic chemotherapy may require blood transfusion. Occasionally, Coombs-positive autoimmune haemolytic anaemia may be found, requiring corticosteroid therapy (p. 69).

The altered host response in the lymphomas and the effects of cytotoxic drugs frequently result in infectious complications. Infections may be poorly localized due to the patient's impaired resistance and septicaemia is not infrequent, requiring intensive antibacterial therapy.

The serum uric acid should be estimated before treatment is begun and, if high, allopurinol 100 mg three times daily given to prevent acute uric acid nephropathy.

The course of the disease depends upon the extent of the disorder, the histological type and the response to therapy; there is great individual variation between the groups and giving a prognosis in an individual case is difficult. Localized benign Hodgkin's disease has an excellent chance of a cure whereas a patient with a disseminated reticulum cell sarcoma will probably succumb within a few weeks or a month. Further consideration of these aspects is given in the individual disorders below.

Follicular lymphoma

Introduction

In follicular lymphoma the neoplastic cells are arranged in a well-marked follicular pattern. Subdivision into reticulum cell, lymphoblastic and lymphocytic cell type is sometimes made and transformation to reticulum cell sarcoma or lymphosarcoma is common. It may occur in one group of glands or in several or in other lymphoid tissue such as the spleen. It comprises about 10% of the lymphomas, has a male to female sex ratio of 2 : 1 and shows an increasing incidence with age.

Clinical features

The usual presenting symptom is related to the presence of a lump. Sometimes this may be found incidentally upon examination of patients presenting with non-specific complaints such as tiredness. The neck is the most common site of lymphadenopathy but other nodes and the spleen may be affected. The condition may remain localized for many years but eventually usually progresses both by extension at the primary site and by involvement of other lymphatic tissues. In the later stages the condition resembles closely the more malignant lymphomas.

Laboratory findings

Laboratory examination of the blood shows no features of note in the early stages. Surgical biopsy of a node or other neoplastic tissue is essential. Enlargement and a follicular structure may be evident macroscopically. Microscopically, large follicles of reticulum cells, lymphoblasts and lymphocytes replace the normal structures. In advanced cases a picture intermediate between this and a reticulum cell sarcoma or lymphosarcoma may be seen.

Diagnosis

The diagnosis, which may be suspected on clinical grounds, is confirmed by histological examination of a biopsy. A similar picture may be found in reactive follicular hyperplasia of the lymph nodes which may occur, for example, in rheumatoid arthritis. A careful assessment of the clinical findings and the opinion of an experienced histologist will usually settle the matter.

Treatment and course

Treatment depends upon the condition of the patient. If the lesion is localized, total excision may be possible but usually radiotherapy is given to the area and is the treatment of choice for local lesions. If the condition is generalized, chemotherapy with an alkylating agent such as cyclophosphamide should be given. The prognosis varies with the stage of the disease but the average survival from diagnosis is about 5 years. Much longer survivals have, however, been recorded and a few patients are cured by radiotherapy or surgery.

Reticulum cell sarcoma

Introduction

A malignant lymphoma, reticulum cell sarcoma is characterized by the destruction of normal lymphoid tissue by sheets of malignant reticulum cells. It resembles lymphosarcoma and Hodgkin's sarcoma but can usually be separated from them histologically. The condition comprises about 20% of the lymphomas, has a male to female ratio of 2 : 1 and shows an increasing incidence with age.

Clinical features

Clinically the usual presenting symptom is the presence of a lump due to lymph node enlargement. The neck is the commonest site but all other nodes may be involved and the spleen may be enlarged. The condition may be localized to start with but rapidly becomes generalized. Involvement of extranodal sites is relatively common and patients may present with lesions in sites such as the stomach or, less often, the small or large intestine or other tissues.

Laboratory findings

Laboratory examination of the blood shows no features of note in the early stages. Surgical biopsy of a lymph node or other affected tissue is necessary for diagnosis. Microscopically, the normal lymphoid tissue is replaced by malignant reticulum cells. Similar cells may be found in the bone marrow and occasionally in the later stages in the blood.

Diagnosis

The diagnosis may be suspected on clinical grounds but histological examination is necessary for confirmation.

Treatment and course

If the condition is localized, surgical excision and radiotherapy may be beneficial. If it is generalized, chemotherapy with an alkylating agent such as cyclophosphamide is recommended. Although a temporary response may occur the disorder soon relapses and becomes resistant to treatment. Most of the patients die within 1 year but a few survive for 5 years. Improved results have been said to follow the combined use of vincristine and cyclophosphamide.

Lymphosarcoma

Introduction

The neoplasm lymphosarcoma is characterized by replacement of normal lymphoid tissue by malignant lymphoblasts and lymphocytes. It may follow follicular lymphoma or arise primarily. In some cases invasion of the blood stream occurs, simulating lymphocytic leukaemia; indeed, the two disorders are closely related. It comprises about 20% of lymphomas, has a male to female ratio of 2 : 1 and an increasing incidence with age.

Clinical features

Most patients present with enlarged lymph nodes, which may occasionally be painful. General malaise and symptoms due to the pressure of enlarged nodes may be present. Involvement of lymphoid tissue elsewhere is not uncommon. There may be tonsillar or nasopharyngeal involvement, hepatosplenomegaly and about 10% of patients will have gastrointestinal involvement at some stage. Lymphosarcoma is the most common lymphoma to involve the small intestine and may cause bleeding, intestinal obstruction, intussusception or malabsorption.

Laboratory findings

Laboratory examination of the blood in the early stages may show no features of note. At a later stage in some cases abnormal lymphoid cells are found in the peripheral blood, These resemble the cells found in chronic lymphocytic leukaemia but are often larger and more pleomorphic. The bone marrow is often infiltrated with such lymphoid cells. Surgical biopsy of a node or other affected tissue is usually necessary for diagnosis. The normal tissue is replaced by sheets of lymphoblasts and lymphocytes, which may also invade the surrounding tissue.

Diagnosis

The diagnosis, which may be suspected on clinical grounds, is usually confirmed by laboratory tests. The blood and bone marrow examination may be diagnostic but a lymph node or other tissue biopsy is usually necessary. Differentiation between chronic lymphocytic leukaemia may be difficult. If the leucocyte count is increased and the percentage of lymphocytes high, the condition is generally regarded as a leukaemia. Histologically, invasion of lymph node capsules is more common in lymphosarcoma but often the two conditions are indistinguishable.

Treatment and course

If the condition is localized, surgical excision and radiotherapy may be given. If generalized, chemotherapy with an alkylating agent such as cyclophosphamide is recommended. The prognosis is generally poor, most patients dying within 2 years; a few, however, survive for 5 or more years. Younger patients generally do badly.

Burkitt's lymphoma

Burkitt's lymphoma resembles a lymphoblastic lymphosarcoma histologically. It differs in its predilection for the jaw bones and ovaries and its geographical distribution which appears to be related to climate. It is found in Africa, New Guinea and Brazil. Less often, tumours with identical histological appearances have been found in the United States and other developed countries. There, the clinical picture is dominated by abdominal tumours. Central nervous system involvement is important in both groups. The Epstein–Barr virus has been found in association with this tumour.

Therapy with a single large dose of cyclophosphamide intravenously often results in prolonged remission.

Hodgkin's disease

Introduction

Hodgkin's disease is a neoplastic proliferation of the reticulum cells and lymphocytes of the lymphoid tissues. It comprises some 50% of the lymphomas, has a male to female ratio of 2 or 3 : 1 and is found at all ages. It can be divided into separate but overlapping types depending upon the natural history and histology.

The classification of Hodgkin's disease on pathological grounds was first proposed by Jackson and Parker and divided into benign paragranuloma, the usual classical granulomatous form, and the more malignant Hodgkin's sarcoma. More recently, a classification into four types has been proposed, called lymphocytic predominance, nodular sclerosis, mixed cellularity and lymphocytic depletion. This is not entirely satisfactory and Cross has recently proposed a further classification divided into reticular, histiocytic and fibroblastic (nodular sclerosing) groups. The unique feature of Hodgkin's disease is the Reed–Sternberg cell (p. 149).

Clinical features

The most usual presentation is with painless enlargement of the lymph nodes, most often cervical and less often axillary, hilar or inguinal. The nodes are characteristically non-tender and discrete, although they may become matted together, and they usually are firm but not stony hard.

Hilar adenopathy may cause bronchial compression and consequent segmental atelectasis. Occasionally, mediastinal gland enlargement leads to superior vena caval obstruction or to recurrent laryngeal nerve palsy. Localized deposits may cause nerve compression elsewhere and paraplegia may develop with epidural tumours.

In more advanced cases, moderate splenomegaly or hepatosplenomegaly may be evident. Jaundice may occur in a few, late in the disease, due to intrahepatic cholestasis. Autoimmune haemolytic anaemia, which occasionally complicates Hodgkin's disease, must also be remembered as a cause of jaundice.

There may be clinical evidence of intra-abdominal disease. Occasionally, infiltration occurs in the wall of the stomach or in the small intestine, which leads to malabsorption. Ascites is sometimes found with intra-abdominal disease, often with more malignant forms of Hodgkin's disease ('Hodgkin's sarcoma').

Bony deposits also may occur and cause severe pain or, less often, pathological fractures.

Systemic symptoms may be present and lead the patient to seek medical attention. These are anorexia, fatigue, weight loss, fever which may be continuous or remittent, pruritus which on occasion is quite intractable and a peculiar phenomenon of pain in affected sites induced by drinking alcohol. Even quite small amounts of alcohol can produce this phenomenon.

Table 10.1. Clinical staging of Hodgkin's disease

Stage	*Location*
I	Disease confined to one anatomical region or to two contiguous regions on the same side of the diaphragm
II	Disease involving more than two contiguous areas or two non-contiguous regions on the same side of the diaphragm
III	Disease on both sides of the diaphragm but limited to lymphatic structures (lymph nodes, spleen, Waldeyer's ring)
IV	Disease which has spread beyond lymphatic structures (e.g. liver, lung, bone marrow, gastrointestinal tract).

Each stage is subclassified:
A: absence of systemic symptoms;
B: presence of systemic symptoms.

Clinical staging

It has been found that patients with Hodgkin's disease limited to one group of lymph nodes have a better prognosis than those whose disease is already disseminated at the time of presentation. The prognosis is also better in the absence of systemic symptoms than when they are present. Not only the prognosis but also the treatment depends on accurate clinical staging. The currently accepted stages are shown in Table 10.1. Patients who are found after full evaluation to be in stages I or II are treated with intensive radiotherapy to both involved and adjacent areas (extended field technique). This approach has significantly increased the cure rate and the duration of remission of this particular group of patients.

Laboratory findings

A mild to moderate anaemia, usually normochromic or slightly hypochromic, may be present and eosinophilia is found in about 15% of cases. Diagnostic cells may be present in smears of bone marrow aspirated from a point of bony tenderness. However, the definitive laboratory test is that of lymph node or other tissue biopsy; the gland shows a destruction of the normal architecture and is replaced by reticular cells, lymphocytes and varying amounts of fibrous tissue, eosinophils, neutrophils and plasma cells. The abnormal reticulum cells may form giant cells; some of these have mirror image nuclei and are known as Reed–Sternberg cells. They have large inclusion-like nucleoli and nuclear polyploidy, in association with an inflammatory cellular proliferation. It is usually a requirement for histological diagnosis; otherwise, conditions such as reactive lymphadenitis may be confused with Hodgkin's disease.

Evaluation of the patient

Once the diagnosis is histologically established by lymph node biopsy, there should be careful evaluation of the patient to assess the extent of tumour involvement. This should include a detailed history and physical examination, urinalysis, complete blood count, chest x-ray with tomography if hilar lymphadenopathy is suspected, skeletal x-ray survey, lymphangiography to assess the possibility of para-aortic lymphadenopathy, liver function tests including radioisotopic liver scan and the appropriate investigation of any localizing complaints. A radioisotopic splenic scan may reveal evidence of focal deposits. A negative scan is not so reliable, however, and because a small percentage of lymphangiograms will be falsely negative in some centres it is customary to perform laparotomy, lymph node biopsies and splenectomy. The place of this procedure as a routine part of the work-up is not yet clearly established, however.

Treatment and course

For patients with stage I and II disease radical radiotherapy is the treatment of choice, usually in a minimum tumour dose of 3,500–4,000 rads over 4–6 weeks. 'Extended field' radiotherapy, which involves the treatment of contiguous areas, recognizes the orderly spread of Hodgkin's disease. This concept has been extended further to 'total nodal' irradiation where all lymph node regions and the splenic area are treated. Not all agree with this approach. Intensive radiotherapy is arduous for the patient and carries the risk of damage to the heart, lungs and kidneys in addition to the complications of bone marrow depression. However, a significant number of prolonged remissions and cures are being obtained with these techniques.

Some have treated stage III A patients with intensive radiotherapy but most use chemotherapy either with single alkylating agents (p. 142) or with a combination of drugs for stages III and IV. The use of drug combinations is designed to make use of the additive effect of drugs with varying modes of action but whose toxic side-effects are not additive, thus permitting greater doses to be used. Significantly greater numbers of remissions, which may be very prolonged, are being obtained. The most commonly used regimen is the MOPP regimen (mustard, Oncovin (vincristine), procarbazine and prednisone). Two-week courses are given every month, if tolerated, for six cycles. This regimen results in morbidity in some patients and it should not be used without adequate laboratory control and facilities for the management of severe marrow aplasia and its consequences.

Localized palliative radiotherapy has a place for patients with stage III and IV disease when local complications such as nerve compression occur.

The course of the disease is extremely variable. If the disease is localized, over half the patients will survive 5 years or more, but if generalized, death usually occurs in 1 or 2 years. Using single agents, unmaintained remissions usually last several months only, but with combination chemotherapy, median remissions of 2 years have been obtained.

Further reading

BODLEY SCOTT, R. (1970). Cancer chemotherapy—the first twenty-five years. *Brit. med. J.* **4**, 259–64.

JOHNSON, R. E. (1970). Modern approaches to the radiotherapy of the lymphomas. *Semin. Hemat.* **6**, 357–75.

ULTMANN, J. E. and NIXON, D. D. (1970). The therapy of lymphoma. *Semin. Hemat.* **6**, 376–403.

11 Thrombopoiesis and its disorders

PLATELET PHYSIOLOGY

The normal integrity of the vascular system depends not only on the blood vessels themselves but also upon tissue damage, plasma factors and thrombocytes. Haemostasis after injury can be divided into two stages; the first is temporary and lasts an hour or so and the second is more permanent.

The first stage involves contraction of the vessel wall and the plugging of the leak with aggregated thrombocytes. Contraction of the vessels is partly controlled by nervous impulses mediated by an axon reflex and partly due to the release of pressor agents by the tissues and thrombocytes. Platelets adhere to the collagen of the injured vessel, then reversibly aggregate due to the release of adenosine diphosphate (release reaction) and subsequently undergo an irreversible change in which they fuse (viscous metamorphosis). Blood released into the tissues may coagulate through the influence of tissue enzymes (extrinsic thromboplastin system).

The second stage of haemostasis involves the production of a thrombus in the vessel at the site of the injury. A variety of factors influence the complex changes involved in the formation of fibrin, filaments of which form around the aggregated thrombocytes. The thrombus thus formed may extend some way along the lumen of the damaged vessel and cells may be enmeshed in its structure. Eventually, healing takes place with organization of the thrombus and possibly recanalization of the vessel.

In this chapter we are concerned with the thrombocytes or platelets which are formed by budding and dissolution of the cytoplasm of mature megakaryocytes in the bone marrow (see Plate 1). The megakaryocytes are formed by the multiplication and maturation of megakaryoblasts, the first recognizable cells of the series. The megakaryoblast differs from the myeloblast in being slightly larger. By a process of nuclear division without cytoplasmic division it passes through a promegakaryocytic stage to the mature megakaryocyte. This giant polyploid cell is prominent in the bone marrow smears and is readily recognized because of its large size; it may be up to 100 μm in diameter. The nucleus is multilobed, the chromatin pattern coarse and there are no nucleoli; the cytoplasm contains masses of purplish-red granules. Occasionally, whole or fragmented megakaryocytes are found in the peripheral blood. The thrombocytes are 2–4 μm in diameter and stain purplish-blue. The factors controlling the maturation of the megakaryocytes and the production of platelets are not fully understood. A humoral factor, thrombopoietin, has been described. About half the thrombocytes survive in the circulation for 5 days and a few survive for up to 10 days before being destroyed. There are no thrombocyte reserves, but they may be sequestrated in the tissues and subsequently return to the blood. Usually there are about 250,000 thrombocytes/μl of blood (but the numbers accepted as normal vary from 150,000 to 400,000/μl). In spite of the lack of a nucleus, thrombocytes are active metabolically, containing polysaccharides and a high concentration of phospholipid. In haemostasis they adhere to the edges of any breaks in the vascular endothelium and aggregate at the site, forming a mechanical plug. Some disintegrate, releasing a vasoconstrictor and a coagulant substance concerned with the formation of a thrombus. The vasoconstrictor substance may be serotonin and that which initiates blood coagulation is called 'lipoid' factor (platelet factor 3). The platelets also act mechanically as a focal point for fibrin formation, forming the basis of the thrombus. *In vitro* this function is reflected in the clot retraction which occurs when clotted blood is incubated at 37°C.

Methods of study

Clinical aspects

Studies of platelet function include a clinical examination and laboratory tests. A personal and family history of excessive bleeding or thrombosis is sought and the type of any bleeding noted; drug taking should be inquired into. The skin and mucous membranes are examined for evidence of haemorrhage. Petechiae are small rounded spots due to capillary haemorrhage; fresh lesions appear pink and older ones brown. Purpura is the name given to more extensive haemorrhages into the skin and mucous membranes. The individual lesions are larger than petechiae and they may coalesce to form confluent areas, giving the general appearance of a rash. Ecchymosis or bruising is a more extensive area of haemorrhage in the subcutaneous tissues; the bruises, at first purple, usually change to brown, green and yellow as the haemoglobin is broken down.

Platelet count

The commonest laboratory test is the examination of a panoptic stained blood film for platelets. If they are seen to be frequent, thrombocytopenia is unlikely; if scanty or apparently increased in numbers, a direct platelet count should be carried out. Platelet morphology can be studied in the blood film for any obvious abnormalities but more specialized tests are usually needed to detect qualitative change.

Platelet survival

Studies of platelet survival are occasionally needed in the diagnosis of thrombocytopenia. The patient's platelets (or donor platelets when the patient's platelet count is low) are labelled with the γ-emitting isotope ^{51}Cr and infused into the subject. Survival is measured and organ surface radioactivity over the spleen, liver and heart measured to determine the site of sequestration. Three patterns are seen. In normal subjects or those with decreased platelet production, a normal recovery and survival of transfused platelets are seen. When there is increased platelet destruction, there is poor recovery and a very short survival. In patients with hypersplenism, intermediate recovery and survival figures are obtained.

Tests of platelet function

Tourniquet tests

This test measures capillary fragility and gives abnormal results in those with thrombocytopenia, in some platelet function defects and in increased capillary fragility. The technique of performing the test varies somewhat in different centres but should be standardized. A sphygmomanometer cuff is inflated over the upper arm to 70 mm Hg for 5 minutes. The forearm is then inspected for petechiae, having first ensured that none were present beforehand. More than 15 petechiae in a 1 cm^2 area is a positive result.

Bleeding time

Defects in number or function of platelets result in a prolongation of the bleeding time. The technique of Ivy gives the most consistent results. A blood pressure cuff is inflated to 40 mm Hg over the forearm. Three 1 mm deep incisions are made with a lancet and the blood wiped away every 30 seconds with filter paper. The time taken for each point to stop bleeding is taken and a mean value obtained.

Clot retraction

This is dependent upon the presence of an adequate number of platelets and can be used as a screening test. Clotted blood in glass tubes is observed in a 37°C water bath over a 4-hour period. Normal retraction begins in 30 minutes.

Platelet adhesiveness

The adhesion of platelets drawn through a column of glass beads, if carried out under carefully controlled conditions, is a useful test of platelet function. Characteristically, adhesiveness is reduced in von Willebrand's disease.

Platelet aggregation

Aggregation of platelets in response to various substances can be measured using the change in optical transmission produced by aggregation in platelet-rich plasma. Adenosine diphosphate (ADP) is used most often. Addition of a small amount causes a biphasic response, the first wave being due to the exogenous ADP; then there is a second wave of aggregation due to the release of endogenous ADP from the platelets. Other substances used include collagen, thrombin and adrenaline. These cause single waves of aggregation.

Other tests

The lipid procoagulant, platelet factor 3, enhances the action of factors X and V in converting prothrombin, and may be measured. Platelets may also be tested by their use in the thromboplastin generation test (p. 177).

DISORDERS OF THROMBOPOIESIS

Disorders of thrombopoiesis are generally reflected by quantitative or qualitative changes in the peripheral blood platelets.

An increased concentration of platelets in the blood is called *thrombocytosis*, which may be physiological or pathological. Two types of pathological thrombocytosis may be distinguished: reactive and thrombocythaemic. The reactive type follows known stimuli and regresses if the stimulus is removed. Thrombocythaemia is part of a progressive malignant process and, whilst rare as a single entity (idiopathic thrombocythaemia), it generally accompanies one of the commoner myeloproliferative disorders, chronic granulocytic leukaemia, myelofibrosis or polycythaemia vera.

A decreased concentration of platelets is called *thrombocytopenia*; if severe, it may be associated with bleeding. It commonly follows other disorders (secondary thrombocytopenia) but in some cases no other disease can be found and the condition is called idiopathic or primary thrombocytopenia.

Qualitative changes in the platelets may be indicated by normal forms in the peripheral blood; large and bizarre shapes are sometimes seen. Abnormality of function (thrombasthenia) may also occur in the absence of other obvious changes.

Thrombocytosis

Reactive thrombocytosis

Increased numbers of functionally normal platelets are found in the blood following haemorrhage, haemolysis, trauma and surgery. The increase may be so great as to be associated with thrombosis; this is particularly likely after splenectomy, and some surgeons give prophylactic anticoagulant therapy post-operatively. Patients who have a persistent non-progressive thrombocytosis for which no stimulus can be found can be said to have idiopathic thrombocytosis.

Thrombocythaemic thrombocytosis

Thrombocytosis may be found at times in any of the myeloproliferative disorders (see Fig. 7.1) and is associated with increased numbers of megakaryocytes in the bone marrow and, in some cases, in other sites such as the spleen as part of the extramedullary haemopoietic process. The abnormality may give rise to thrombosis or haemorrhage or both and occurs not infrequently in chronic granulocytic leukaemia, myelofibrosis and polycythaemia vera. Sometimes the megakaryocyte and platelet increases are so marked as to be the principal feature and in these cases the diagnosis of idiopathic thrombocythaemia (megakaryocytic myelosis) can be made. Some such cases progress to show features of one of the other myeloproliferative syndromes. Another synonym for this condition is haemorrhagic thrombocythaemia, since many present as a bleeding disorder, the site of bleeding usually being the gastrointestinal tract. The platelets are increased in number and may be morphologically and functionally normal. Hypochromic anaemia is very frequently present since bleeding is often severe but there may also be a slight erythrocytosis and, in many, there is usually a moderate leucocytosis. On occasion it may be difficult to distinguish this condition from reactive thrombocytosis secondary to gastrointestinal haemorrhage. Frequently in idiopathic thrombocythaemia there is splenomegaly, however, and the bone marrow findings usually show a more striking megakaryocytic hyperplasia. Laparotomy for the bleeding is hazardous in these patients because the poor platelet function results in uncontrolled operative oozing. If the spleen is removed during the operation, the platelet count usually increases to uncontrollable levels post-operatively, causing both thrombotic and haemorrhagic complications. The treatment of these disorders is that of the underlying condition; the platelet count can usually be reduced by radiation with ^{32}P or by giving busulphan. If these are ineffective a trial with phenylalanine mustard (melphalan) is worth considering and recently thrombocytopheresis has been advocated as a means of rapidly controlling the platelet count.

Thrombocytopenia

Thrombocytopenia may be primary (idiopathic) or secondary to a wide variety of conditions. Two general groups can be distinguished: those in which the megakaryocytes in the bone marrow are decreased with depressed platelet production and those in which the megakaryocytes are present in normal or increased numbers, indicating normal or increased platelet production but with increased peripheral destruction of platelets.

Thrombocytopenia with decreased platelet production

Thrombocytopenia with decreased platelet production may be part of a generalized depression of the bone marrow (hypoplastic or aplastic anaemia) or present by itself. It is found in diffuse bone marrow diseases such as leukaemias, lymphomas, myeloma, secondary carcinomatosis, poisoning by chemicals or drugs and following ionizing radiation. Alcoholics are frequently found to be moderately severely thrombocytopenic following a bout of drinking. Withdrawal of alcohol results in a rapid return of the platelet count to normal. Thrombocytopenia has been produced in healthy volunteers given alcohol.

Thrombocytopenia with increased platelet production

Thombocytopenia with increased platelet production is found when there is excessive destruction or dilution of the platelets in the circulation. The presence of megakaryocytic hyperplasia is common.

With massive transfusion for profuse haemorrhage or with exchange transfusion, thrombocytopenia usually occurs due to dilution especially if the donor blood is not fresh.

Destruction of platelets may be due to immunological or other factors. Conditions associated with this type of thrombocytopenia include transfusions, drug and toxin sensitivity, disseminated intravascular coagulation, various infections, neonatal thrombocytopenia, systemic lupus erythematosus and 'hypersplenism'. It may also be associated with haemolytic anaemia or with neutropenia. In many there is no evident cause and this group is said to have idiopathic thrombocytopenic purpura (see below).

Drug and toxin sensitivity

In cases of sensitivity, the drug, usually apronal (Sedormid), quinine' quinidine, digitoxin or a barbiturate, acts as a hapten causing an antibody to be developed against the platelet–drug complex. The condition remits when the drug is stopped. Sensitivity to the drug may be demonstrated by a 'patch' test on the skin; purpura develops under the patch in sensitive persons and may be due to sensitivity on the part of the capillary which shares a common antigen with the platelets. This test should only be carried out after due consideration because it may precipitate a more intense thrombocytopenia. *In vitro* tests of platelet agglutination, lysis or complement fixation in the presence of the drug may be positive. If all these tests are negative, the drug may be still responsible and a small test dose can be given and the platelet count followed to further the diagnosis. This also may be dangerous, leading to further bleeding, and should only be carried out after very careful consideration of all the factors involved.

Infections

Thrombocytopenia may occur during the acute or convalescent stages in a wide variety of infections. The most common are viral and include respiratory infections, measles, infectious mononucleosis, chickenpox, mumps and hepatitis. Consumption of platelets, causing thrombocytopenia in disseminated intravascular coagulation associated with severe infections, is becoming recognized more frequently.

Neonatal thrombocytopenia

In neonatal thrombocytopenia the newborn baby's thrombocytopenia is due to maternal antibodies in the baby's circulation. It remits spontaneously as the antibody disappears with time.

Systemic lupus erythematosus

Systemic lupus erythematosus may be associated with thrombocytopenia. LE cells should be sought in any case of thrombocytopenia without another obvious cause. The mechanism of the thrombocytopenia is the formation of an antibody against the patient's platelets.

Hypersplenism

Enlargement of the spleen, or even overactivity without enlargement, may result in a thrombocytopenia, either singly or as part of a pancytopenia. This is due to sequestration of the thrombocytes by the spleen. Splenectomy usually results in a remission.

Miscellaneous

Antibody formation may occur against the three main cellular components of the blood, either individually or together. Thrombocytopenia may therefore be present but relatively less important in autoimmune haemolytic anaemias and in immune neutropenias. Thrombocytopenia due to mechanical destruction may occur in extracorporeal circulation of the blood. Platelets are often depressed in disorders of folic acid and cobalamin metabolism; for example, pernicious anaemia sometimes presents with haemorrhagic manifestations due to thrombocytopenia.

Insect and snake venoms may also cause thrombocytopenia. Uraemia may be associated with defective platelet function and in some cases there is thrombocytopenia. There is some evidence of platelet dysfunction in von Willebrand's disease, which is considered in Chapter 12.

Idiopathic thrombocytopenia purpura (ITP)

In some cases, the cause of thrombocytopenia remains undetermined in spite of all investigations; such cases are called idiopathic or primary. Most patients are children or young adults. An acute type, developing within a few days, is more common in children and may cause serious loss of blood; a chronic type, presenting with recurrent crops of purpura, is usually less severe. Platelet antibodies can be demonstrated in about 60% of cases. Platelets infused into such patients have a reduced survival (1 or 2 hours, compared with the normal mean of 5 days). Usually there is megakaryocytic hyperplasia but this is not invariable.

Clinical features of thrombocytopenia

The patient with thrombocytopenia usually presents with bruises and bleeding due to the platelet defect or with symptoms referable to an underlying disorder. Sometimes the condition may be discovered incidentally, on laboratory examination, without causing symptoms or signs. Thrombocytopenia may develop insidiously or acutely; bruising and bleeding are usually present if the platelet concentration is below 50,000/μl of blood, but there is no exact correlation between platelet concentration and haemorrhage. Sometimes patients with less than 10,000/μl show no bleeding tendency unless exposed to trauma; the vessels, and possibly other factors, as well as the platelets are obviously important. Bleeding is usually present as petechiae in the skin, the mucous membranes and conjunctivae and may give rise to haematuria, epistaxis and melaena. Deep tissue bleeding is usually more serious; haemorrhage in the eye may lead to loss of vision, and in the nervous system to the clinical picture of cerebral haemorrhage, a common cause of death in thrombocytopenia. Splenomegaly is usually absent in idiopathic cases; if present, the condition is probably secondary to some other disorder. Thrombocytopenia may remit spontaneously and acute forms may become chronic. The prognosis depends upon the underlying disorder, if any, and the response to treatment.

Laboratory examination

Thrombocytopenia is present, platelets being scanty or absent in the blood smear. Counts below 50,000/μl are usual; counts below 10,000 are inaccurate and are best recorded as 'less than 10,000 platelets/μl of blood present'. Depending upon the underlying disorder, there may be anaemia and leucopenia. The bone marrow shows a variable picture with regard to the megakaryocytes, which may be absent, normal or hyperplastic; there may be a shift to the left in the maturation pattern of the megakaryocytes with a preponderance of immature forms.

Other tests which may be performed include those for bleeding time and clot retraction; the capillary fragility test should be carried out if there is no obvious purpura. In some centres tests for platelet agglutination can be made and if a drug is suspected, its effect upon platelets assessed. The radioisotopic platelet survival in ITP will show both a poor recovery of infused platelets and a short half-life which is often reduced to 1–2 hours. Surface counting over the spleen and liver is used to assess the site of destruction of platelets.

Treatment

Treatment of secondary thrombocytopenia depends upon the cause. For example, any toxic agents should be withdrawn and any underlying disease treated along the usual lines.

If this is not successful or the condition is idiopathic and the patient's life is in danger from bleeding, as it frequently is in the acute stage, corticosteroids should be given. High doses (50–100 mg of prednisone per day) should be used at first and then gradually reduced after improvement occurs. If an improvement is not seen within 3 weeks or if it cannot be maintained when the dosage is reduced, as is often the case in chronic cases, splenectomy is performed. This results in a clinical cure in 70–80% of the cases but there is an appreciable mortality. Some clinicians advise splenectomy first and only if this fails do they use corticosteroids. There is some evidence to suggest that the spleen may be an important site of antiplatelet antibody synthesis in ITP, but it is generally believed that the principal effect of splenectomy is the removal of a 'filter' which is trapping antibody-coated platelets. Long-continued corticosteroid therapy is undesirable and should only be used with patients whose thrombocytopenia has not been corrected by splenectomy. In such cases, repeated attempts at lessening the dosage of drug should be made. Some such patients benefit from immunosuppressive therapy with cyclophosphamide. This is not usually of use in the acute stage and it may take weeks before a remission is induced.

In an emergency, platelet transfusions may be given but the antibody present in ITP usually results in rapid destruction of infused platelets and, therefore, lack of clinical effectiveness. Platelet transfusions are often effective when the thrombocytopenia is not of immunological origin. However, with repeated blood or platelet transfusions, antibodies frequently develop so that infused platelets become progressively less effective.

Disorders of platelet function

A number of congenital and acquired defects of platelet function have been described. The terminology is confusing but there are two fundamental defects—a lack of response to ADP (thrombasthenia) and an abnormal release reaction (thrombocytopathy or thrombopathy).

Thrombasthenia (Glanzmann's disease) is a hereditary bleeding disorder where a prolonged bleeding time, poor clot retraction and failure *in vitro* of platelets to aggregate when ADP, collagen, serotonin or adrenaline are added.

An *abnormal release reaction* may be associated with bleeding in a heterogeneous group of congenital and acquired disorders. Acquired disturbances may be seen in renal disease, liver disease and following ingestion of certain drugs, notably aspirin. Following its ingestion, the secondary wave of aggregation in response to ADP does not occur, due to the failure of release of intrinsic ADP. As little as 150 mg of aspirin in one dose may have this effect for up to a week. The bleeding time of normal individuals is slightly increased by aspirin but a much greater prolongation may be seen in severe haemophiliacs, in von Willebrand's disease and during anticoagulant therapy. Other drugs with similar effects include phenylbutazone, glyceryl guaiacolate, sulphinpyrazone and dipyridamole.

Further reading

BALDINI, MARIO G. (1972). Idiopathic thrombocytopenic purpura and the ITP syndrome. *Med. Clin. N. Amer.* **56**, 47–64.

GYNN, T. N., MESSMORE, H. L. and FRIEDMAN, I. A. (1972). Drug-induced thrombocytopenia. *Med. Clin. N. Amer.* **56**, 65–79.

TURPIE, A. G. G., MCNICOL, G. P. and DOUGLAS, A. S. (1971). Platelets: haemostasis and thrombosis. In: *Recent Advances in Haematology*, 249–301. Ed. A. Goldberg and M. C. Brain. Churchill Livingstone, Edinburgh and London.

12 Haemostasis and its disorders

NORMAL HAEMOSTASIS

The spontaneous arrest of haemorrhage following injury depends upon a variety of factors which include the blood vessels themselves, the platelets, plasma factors and the damaged tissues. Haemostasis, as it is called, can be divided into two stages, the first being temporary and lasting an hour or two and the second permanent. The first stage involves contraction of the vessel wall and the plugging of the leak with aggregated platelets. Contraction of the vessels is partly controlled by nervous impulses mediated by an axon reflex and partly due to the release of pressor agents such as serotonin by the tissues and platelets. Platelets first adhere to the exposed subendothelial collagen fibres of the torn vessel, then reversibly aggregate associated with the release of ADP, forming a loose voluminous aggregate which is still permeable to the bloodstream. Transformation into an impermeable plug then occurs under the influence of thrombin.

The second stage of haemostasis involves the production of a thrombus in the vessel at the site of the injury. A variety of factors influence the complex changes involved in the formation of fibrin, filaments of which form around the aggregated platelets. The role of plasma factors in haemostasis is discussed in Chapter 13. The thrombus thus formed may extend some way along the lumen of the damaged vessel and cells may be enmeshed in its structure. Eventually healing takes place with organization of the thrombus and possibly recanalization of the vessel.

DISORDERS OF HAEMOSTASIS

A haemorrhagic state may result from defects of the blood vessels, the platelets or the plasma factors, either singly or in combination. Disorders of the platelets have already been described (Chapter 11). Blood vessel defects are considered here and plasma factors in Chapter 13.

The most important investigation in assessing the likely cause of a bleeding diathesis is the history. This should include details about any purpuric or haemorrhagic episode, including the age at onset, the severity and length and the necessity for transfusions. A general medical history with particular note of liver disease, drugs and all operations, including dental procedures, is needed. A family history should be taken and if positive the possible mode of inheritance determined. From this and the clinical examination, the type of tests required will be determined. These usually include a capillary fragility test (in the absence of obvious purpura), platelet count, bleeding time, coagulation time, prothrombin time and thromboplastin generation screening test (for activated partial thromboplastin time). Details of these tests are given on pp. 152 and 175.

Blood vessel defects

Introduction

Disorders of the blood vessels generally cause purpura and bleeding from mucous membranes or, following trauma, rather than extensive bruising and joint and deep tissue haemorrhages. They are divided into the acquired and the congenital disorders in which there is often a history of onset at an early age and a positive family history.

Acquired defects may be due to allergic vasculitis or secondary to a variety of factors (infections, drugs, dysproteinaemias, ascorbic acid deficiency and old age).

The congenital defects include von Willebrand's disease, hereditary haemorrhagic telangiectasia and Ehlers–Danlos syndrome.

Methods of study

The methods used in the study of the blood vessels and capillaries include the capillary fragility test and the bleeding time. It is usual to test platelet function at the same time (p. 153), because some of the disorders involve both capillaries and platelets and in some conditions plasma factors are also defective. Rarely, biopsy of a piece of skin or muscle is required so that the vessels may be examined histologically.

Allergic disorders of the blood vessels

A miscellaneous group of disorders associated with bruising and purpura are thought to be due to allergic or hypersensitivity reactions occurring in small vessel walls. These are called the allergic vasculitides and comprise variants including anaphylactoid purpura (Henoch–Schönlein purpura) and systemic disorders such as systemic lupus erythematosus and polyarteritis nodosa.

Anaphylactoid purpura

Anaphylactoid purpura is generalized arteriolitis and is due to a hypersensitivity reaction. The resultant increase in vascular permeability causes haemorrhages into subcutaneous and other tissues. It resembles rheumatic fever and glomerulonephritis in that it frequently follows a streptococcal infection but other bacterial allergens can sometimes be found.

Clinical features

The disorder is found more frequently in children and often follows a week or two after a sore throat or similar mild upper respiratory infection. A purpuric rash often with larger haemorrhagic spots and raised areas is present, usually over the back and limbs. Repeated crops of spots may occur and so lesions at different stages of development may be seen together. Abdominal pain, sometimes accompanied by vomiting, diarrhoea and intestinal haemorrhage is frequently found due to vasculitis in the intestinal wall. Occasionally, intussusception or perforation complicates the picture. In many cases polyarthritis is also present and, in others, haematuria. The most important systemic lesions are found in the kidneys in nearly half of all patients. Haematuria may be either microscopic or macroscopic and proteinuria is common. Histologically there may be focal or a diffuse proliferative glomerulonephritis. The majority of patients fully recover but some continue to have prolonged haematuria and proteinuria without evidence of progression and a few develop progressive chronic renal failure.

Blood picture

The platelet count is normal or only slightly lowered. The capillary fragility test may be positive but the bleeding time is usually normal. Anti-streptococcal antibodies may be present in high titre in the serum.

Treatment

Any infection or other underlying disorder is treated conventionally. The purpura is usually self-limiting and requires no specific treatment. Occasionally, corticosteroid or immunosuppressive therapy is given and while there is usually symptomatic improvement in the articular and gastro-intestinal manifestations, the evidence for a beneficial effect on the renal disease is controversial.

Symptomatic vascular purpuras

In the symptomatic vascular purpuras the platelet count is usually normal although a slight thrombocytopenia may be present. The tourniquet test is frequently positive but the bleeding time is usually normal.

Infections

In infections such as the enteric fevers, endocarditis, meningococcal and other septicaemias, purpura may be due to embolism or toxaemia. It also occurs in some rickettsial and viral diseases, such as infectious mononucleosis, haemorrhagic fever and the exanthemata and appears to be caused by a toxic effect on capillary endothelium. In some cases it appears to represent a hypersensitivity reaction; some of the drugs which can cause an allergic type of thrombocytopenia can also cause this type of purpura. They include many of the common antibiotics, especially ampicillin, sedatives, analgesics and antirheumatic drugs. Withdrawal of the drug usually leads to remission within a few days. A subsequent skin patch test (p. 156) may show the relationship between a drug and the reaction.

Dysproteinaemias

Hyperglobulinaemia, myelomatosis, macroglobulinaemia, cryoglobulinaemia and amyloidosis are all protein anomalies which may be associated with purpura. The mechanism by which the purpura is produced is obscure. However, it has been shown that the abnormal protein can coat the platelets and cause platelet dysfunction. Treatment is that of the underlying condition; corticosteroids may be tried if the purpura is severe.

Other purpuras

In severe ascorbic acid deficiency (scurvy), purpura is thought to be due to fragility of the capillary walls, although platelet dysfunction may also play a part. Large haemorrhages into the soft tissue as well as petechiae may occur.

Senile purpura is common in old people with loose skin on the back of the hands and is due to the loss of support for the capillaries by the connective tissue. The extravasated blood is only slowly absorbed. Purpura may also occur in metabolic disorders such as uraemia, diabetes mellitus and hyperadrenocorticoidism and in fat embolism.

Von Willebrand's disease

Also called pseudohaemophilia, von Willebrand's disease is characterized by an abnormal bleeding tendency, predominantly involving mucosal surfaces. It was thought to be due to a defective contractility of the small arterioles but platelet dysfunction appears to be important and plasma deficiencies occur in some cases. Recently it has been found that a labile plasma factor may correct the bleeding time, and lack of this factor and its effect on platelets may be the fundamental defect. It is a difficult disease to classify and is described here for convenience.

The condition is inherited as an autosomal dominant character and affects both sexes. It varies in severity but bleeding following operation or injury is characteristic; spontaneous bleeding and menorrhagia may also occur. Purpura is not common; the tourniquet test may be either positive or negative. The bleeding time is usually prolonged but may approach normal depending on the site and whether or not the patient is in a bleeding phase. Aspirin has been found to markedly prolong the bleeding time in these patients, a dose of 600 mg being sufficient. Sodium salicylate is without this effect. The platelets are usually normal in numbers but platelet adhesiveness is frequently reduced. Other tests of platelet function are usually normal. Factor VIII may be depressed but not usually to the low levels found in classical haemophilia. The variability of abnormalities has suggested to some that the name von Willebrand's disease may include a heterogeneous group of disorders.

Whole fresh blood, fresh plasma or AHG concentrates are given as required during a bleeding episode and are effective in lessening haemorrhage. Usually 2–4 units of plasma or cryoprecipitate once daily are adequate treatment and reduce a prolonged bleeding time to normal. A rise in the factor VIII level is seen also and is greater and more prolonged than would be expected from the infused factor VIII. After infusion, the patient's factor VIII plasma level continues to rise for 6–12 hours and then falls slowly. Aspirin should be avoided since it makes the bleeding tendency worse.

Hereditary haemorrhagic telangiectasia

Hereditary haemorrhagic telangiectasia is characterized by the presence of numerous telangiectatic dilated arterioles and capillaries in the skin and mucous membranes of the upper respiratory tract and alimentary canal. The condition, which is uncommon, is inherited as an autosomal dominant character.

Bleeding is associated with the abnormal contractility of the small vessels, which are thin and fragile. The telangiectatic spots, which vary in size from 1 mm up to 100 mm in diameter, become more prominent as the patient gets older. Bleeding, which is the predominant feature, may not be marked until adult life. Epistaxes, mouth bleeds and intestinal haemorrhages are the most troublesome. Bleeding from the skin is not usually severe unless traumatized. The blood picture is usually that of an iron deficiency anaemia following haemorrhage. The bleeding time tourniquet test, platelets and coagulation test are all normal.

There is no specific treatment; blood transfusions and iron therapy are given as indicated. If the patient is severely incapacitated by the disorder, a trial of oestrogen therapy may be given but is usually ineffective.

Ehlers–Danlos disease

Ehlers–Danlos disease is a rare hereditary disorder of connective tissue. The blood vessels are unduly fragile, the skin has abnormal elasticity and the joints are hyperextensible. It is transmitted as an autosomal dominant character and is of variable severity. Bruising is common and bleeding is likely following trauma or surgery. There is no specific treatment and trauma or operations must be avoided wherever possible.

Further reading

BEAN, W. B. (1958). *Vascular Spiders and Related Lesions of the Skin.* Charles C Thomas, Springfield, Illinois.

MURPHY, E. A. and SALZMAN, E. W. (1972). The diagnosis of von Willebrand's disease. *Blood* **39**, 284–7.

STORMARKER, H. and OWREN, P. A. (1971). Physiopathology of haemostasis. *Semin. Hemat.* **8**, 3–29.

WEISS, H. J. (1968). Von Willebrand's disease—diagnostic criteria. *Blood* **32** 668–79.

13 Plasma factors in haemostasis

Introduction

Plasma contributes to haemostasis in coagulation and in fibrinolysis. The formation of a stable intravascular thrombus depends upon the conversion of the soluble plasma protein, fibrinogen, into a fibrin clot. A similar mechanism occurs when blood clots outside the body, and the various theories of blood coagulation are based largely upon *in vitro* tests. The exact relevance of these to intravascular clotting is not always certain but they are of great value in the diagnosis and classification of most of the bleeding disorders.

In the blood there are factors promoting coagulation, factors inhibiting it and factors which dissolve precipitated fibrin. Normally these are held in careful balance. In injury, coagulation factors are beneficial in restricting blood loss but in pathological thrombosis they may be harmful. Anticoagulant factors are helpful in preventing intravascular thrombosis from occurring normally but, if present in excess, may promote haemorrhage.

Similarly, fibrinolytic activity is helpful in removing deposited fibrin after thrombosis but, if pathologically overactive, may cause haemorrhage.

A number of factors are required for coagulation and they can be divided into two systems: the extrinsic or tissue system and the intrinsic or blood system. Activity of either of these systems results in the production of a thromboplastin. This, in the presence of calcium ions, catalyses the reaction which converts prothrombin to thrombin. In its turn, thrombin, in the presence of calcium ions, catalyses the conversion of fibrinogen to fibrin. The sequence of events which occurs during the formation of a thrombus has been characterized by Macfarlane as a 'coagulation cascade' of six enzyme reactions (Fig. 13.1).

Because of the many synonyms which have been used, an International Committee has identified the established factors by roman numerals. The factors which go to make up the extrinsic system are tissue thromboplastin, factor VII, factor X, factor V and factor IV (calcium ions) (Table 13.1). The factors which go to make up the intrinsic system are a wettable surface, factor XII, factor XI, platelet factors, factor VIII, factor IX, factor X, factor V and factor IV (Table 13.2). The individual factors are discussed later in this chapter.

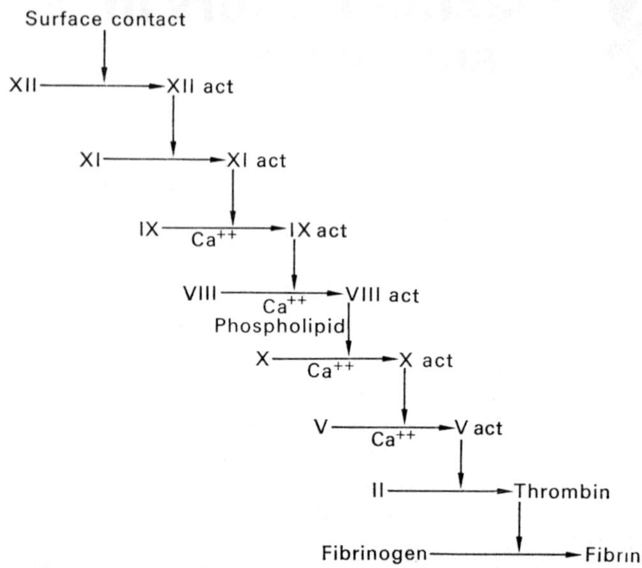

Fig. 13.1. The cascade or waterfall sequence of coagulation.

Table 13.1. Blood coagulation: extrinsic system

Recommended name	*Synonyms*
Tissue thromboplastin (III)	
Factor VII	Stable factor, proconvertin
Factor X	Stuart factor, Prower factor
Factor V	Labile factor, proaccelerin
Factor IV	Calcium ions

Factor VII takes part only in the extrinsic system
Factors VIII, IX and XII take part only in the intrinsic system
Factors IV, V and X are common to both the intrinsic and the extrinsic systems

An alternative to the cascade theory is a system of three enzyme complexes (Fig. 13.2). In the first, factors XII and XI form an activator complex when exposed to certain surfaces such as collagen; this complex, in the presence of calcium ions, then activates factor IX.

The second complex is formed by the interaction of activated factor IX,

Table 13.2. Blood coagulation: intrinsic system

Recommended name	*Synonyms*
Factor XII	Hageman factor, contact factor, surface factor
Factor XI	Plasma thromboplastic antecedent
Platelet factor 3	Includes phospholipids
Factor VIII	Antihaemophilic globulin, antihaemophilic factor
Factor IX	Christmas factor, plasma thromboplastic component
Factor X	Stuart factor, Prower factor
Factor V	Labile factor, proaccelerin
Factor IV	Calcium ions

Factors XI, XII, VIII, IX take part only in the intrinsic system
Factor VII takes part only in the extrinsic system
Factors IV, V and X are common to both the intrinsic and the extrinsic systems

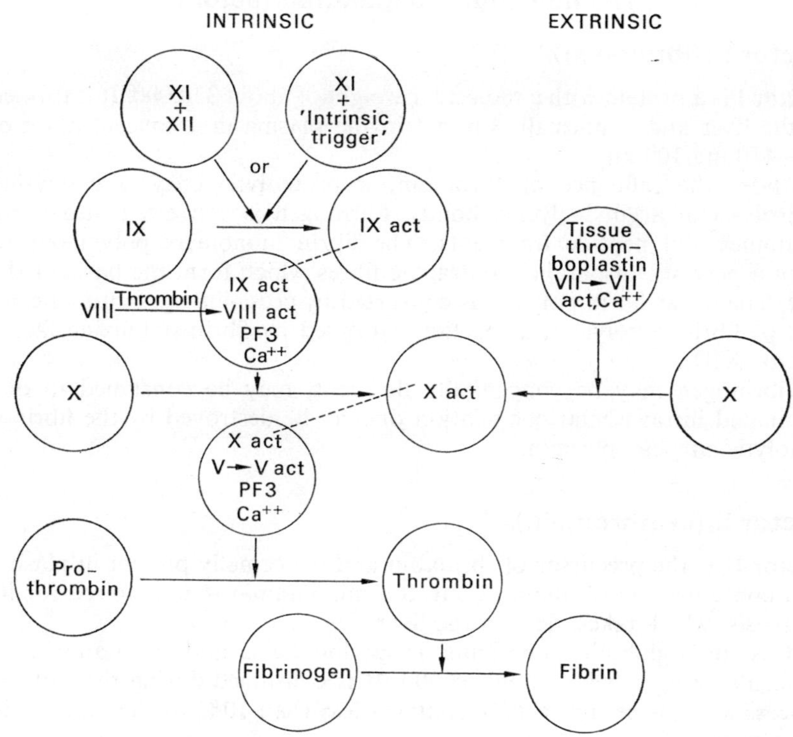

Fig. 13.2. Extrinsic and intrinsic coagulation.

factor VIII, platelet phospholipid (platelet factor 3) and calcium ions to activate factor X. Factor VIII is preactivated by thrombin. In the extrinsic system, an enzyme or enzymes in the microsomal fraction of many tissues, called tissue thromboplastin, together with activated factor VII and calcium ions form a complex which also activates factor X.

In the third sequence, both the extrinsic and intrinsic systems follow a common pathway. A complex is formed with activated factor X, factor V, platelet factor 3 and calcium ions, which converts prothrombin to thrombin. Thrombin then converts fibrinogen to fibrin, which is stabilized under the influence of activated factor XIII (fibrin-stabilizing factor), a transamidase formed from an inactive precursor by the action of thrombin.

What actually initiates coagulation physiologically is poorly understood. Factor XI and a hydrophobic surface activator (perhaps platelet microtubules) are required but factor XII does not seem to be required *in vivo.*

Both extrinsic and intrinsic coagulation systems are necessary for normal haemostasis but their interrelationship is not fully understood.

The individual coagulation factors

Factor I (fibrinogen)

Factor I is a protein with a molecular weight of about 330,000. It is formed in the liver and is normally present in the plasma in a concentration of 250–450 mg/100 ml.

Under the influence of thrombin, a proteolytic enzyme catalysing hydrolysis of arginyl–glycine bonds, fibrinogen is converted into fibrin monomer and peptide fragments. The fibrin monomers polymerize to form a network of parallel contractile fibres which form the basis of the clot. The linear fibrin polymer is converted by cross-linkages into a firmer clot of fibrin copolymer, a reaction catalysed by fibrin-stabilizing factor (factor XIII).

Fibrinogen may be congenitally deficient, may be consumed in disseminated intravascular coagulation or may be destroyed by the fibrinogenolytic enzyme, plasmin.

Factor II (prothrombin)

Factor II is the precursor of thrombin and is normally present in plasma in a concentration of about 10 mg/100 ml. Vitamin K is required for its synthesis, which takes place in the liver.

It is an α-globulin containing 18 amino acids and hexosamine, its molecular weight being about 68,000. It is consumed during the clotting process and the serum usually contains less than 10% of the amount in the plasma.

Congenital hypoprothrombinaemia is rare but an acquired deficiency may occur in hepatic disease, avitaminosis K and, most frequently, following anticoagulant therapy with drugs of the coumarin or indandione classes which inhibit its synthesis.

Factor III (thromboplastin, prothrombin conversion factor)

Thromboplastin has been used as a general term for substances which hasten the clotting of blood. Tissue thromboplastins produced by tissue damage are needed in the extrinsic system and blood thromboplastins in the intrinsic system. It is suggested that the complex of activated factor X, factor V, phospholipid and calcium is the actual prothrombin conversion factor (see Fig. 13.2). The term thromboplastin, therefore, should be avoided, but its use is so widespread that it will probably continue to be used for some time.

Thrombin

Thrombin is a powerful enzyme and is not normally present in blood but is the activated form of prothrombin. Once formed, the molecule has a very short life span. It has a similar composition to prothrombin but is smaller with a molecular weight of about 32,000. It catalyses the conversion of fibrinogen to fibrin. Additionally, thrombin has other actions. Under the influence of thrombin, platelets become fused in the process of viscous metamorphosis. It activates factors VIII and V and converts factor XIII from an inactive to an active form. A unit of thrombin is defined as that amount necessary to clot 1 ml of a standard fibrinogen solution in 15 seconds at 28°C. Partially purified preparations of thrombin are available commercially.

Factor IV (calcium)

Calcium ions are essential for the normal action of thromboplastin and thrombin and many anticoagulants act by binding them. Clinically, deficiencies sufficient to affect the clotting mechanisms probably do not occur since such a degree of hypocalcaemia is incompatible with life.

Factor V

Factor V is called labile factor, plasma accelerator globulin and proaccelerin. It is an unstable protein present in plasma. It accelerates prothrombin conversion and is needed in both the extrinsic and the intrinsic systems. Rare congenital deficiencies have been reported. The plasma concentration may also be low in parenchymal liver disease.

Factor VI

The name factor VI is no longer used; it was given to a factor thought to be activated factor V.

Factor VII

Factor VII is a protein present in plasma, which is relatively stable and present also in serum. It is necessary for the activation of tissue thromboplastin. Congenital deficiencies have been reported and lowered plasma levels occur in liver disease, following oral anticoagulant therapy and in avitaminosis K.

Factor VIII

Factor VIII is also known as antihaemophilic globulin (AHG) and antihaemophilic factor (AHF). It is thought to be a globulin protein of high molecular weight, present in low concentrations (about 12 μg/100 ml) in normal plasma. Although large, it may cross the placental barrier. Electrophoretically it migrates with β-globulin. After assay, the plasma values are expressed as a percentage of the mode of normal people and the range is 60–200% (or 60–200 units/100 ml) (see Table 13.3). Its source is unknown but some think it is synthesized in the reticular system. The spleen is a rich source of factor VIII. Unstable on ordinary storage, it can be concentrated by fractionation of plasma and stored in the lyophilized state. *In vivo* it has a half-life of 10–20 hours. Congenital deficiency of the factor is found in classical haemophilia which is inherited as a sex-linked recessive character (p. 180).

Factor IX

Factor IX is also known as plasma thromboplastin component or Christmas factor. It is a plasma globulin of molecular weight about 86,000, also present in serum and fairly stable on storage. Congenital deficiency of the factor is found in haemophilia B (Christmas disease) which is inherited as a sex-linked recessive character (p. 180). Acquired deficiency may be seen in liver disease.

Factor X

Factor X is also known as the Prower factor or Stuart factor. Its exact nature is not known but it is stable and is present in serum as well as in plasma. Congenital deficiencies of the factor are found and the disorder appears to be inherited as an autosomal incompletely recessive character, which is highly penetrant. Acquired deficiencies are found in liver disease and in anticoagulant therapy.

Platelets

Platelets form part of the intrinsic system of coagulation in addition to the mechanical role they play in haemostasis. The substance active in coagulation is made available after platelet aggregation and is called platelet factor 3. Recent evidence suggests that another platelet factor (platelet factor 4) may be important in the aggregation and precipitation of fibrinogen and its derivatives. After coagulation has occurred the platelets take part in clot retraction.

Factor XI

Factor XI, which is also called plasma thromboplastin antecedent, is found in plasma and is probably a protein. It is stable and is present in serum and in plasma which has been absorbed with an aluminium hydroxide gel. Congenital deficiency of the factor is occasionally found, usually in Jews, inherited as an autosomal dominant character.

Factor XII

Factor XII, which is also called the Hageman or contact factor, is probably a protein. Blood deficient in this factor does not clot in the normal time in the test-tube; however, the patients from whom the blood is taken have no bleeding tendency. The physiological role of this factor is uncertain but it is absorbed on to rough surfaces, hence the name contact factor.

Factor XIII

Also known as fibrin-stabilizing factor, factor XIII cross-links soluble polymerized fibrin which then becomes stabilized as insoluble fibrin.

Congenital deficiency of factor XIII is very rare and is inherited in an autosomal recessive manner. The clinical picture is characteristic with neonatal umbilical haemorrhage, intracranial haemorrhage, excessive secondary bleeding from wounds and poor wound healing.

Haemorrhagic disease due to acquired factor XIII deficiency has not yet been reported. However, low levels have been described in liver disease, leukaemia and untreated pernicious anaemia.

Anticoagulants

Many of the reactions in normal blood coagulation are thought to be inhibited by physiological anticoagulants which remove or neutralize the coagulant factors. These include antithromboplastin and antithrombin substances. One of these may be heparin but its role in human physiology is uncertain. When given in treatment it inhibits the formation of thromboplastin as well as acting as an antithrombin. A more important physiological antithrombin, designated antithrombin 3, both inactivates thrombin directly and is a cofactor for inactivation by heparin.

Pathological anticoagulants active against coagulation factors may develop on occasion. There are three main classes: those which inactivate factor VIII, those found in patients with systemic lupus erythematosus and a miscellaneous group of substances affecting various other clotting factors. Pathological anticoagulants frequently are antibodies.

Antibodies to factor VIII may develop in haemophiliacs (p. 182) and also sometimes in other patients. They arise in the elderly, in women after childbirth and in patients with a heterogeneous group of conditions of allergic or immune origin. In these, the antibodies arise apparently spontaneously and usually do not increase greatly in titre following transfusion. They often gradually disappear over a period of time. In haemophiliacs, however, the titre often rises after infusion of the substances containing AHG and the antibodies persist.

In systemic lupus erythematosus an anticoagulant may develop which blocks the conversion of prothrombin to thrombin by the activating complex.

The fibrinolytic system

Whilst the formation of the fibrin clot is basic to the haemostatic integrity of the vascular system, the fibrinolytic system is equally important since it maintains its patency. It is also important in keeping patent other structures such as lymphatic vessels, tear ducts and ducts of exocrine glands. Normally, both the coagulation and the fibrinolytic systems are carefully balanced.

A proteolytic enzyme, plasmin, which lyses fibrin but also fibrinogen and factors V and VIII, is normally present in the blood as an inactive precursor, plasminogen (Fig. 13.3). Plasminogen can be activated by direct or indirect activators. Tissue injury may release direct activator, and another direct activator which is present in urine, urokinase, has been used therapeutically. Indirect activation results from the activation of a proactivator which is probably part of the plasminogen molecule. Activators may be released by various tissues, especially veins. Streptokinase, isolated from a streptococcal culture, has been used therapeutically to cause thrombolysis and activates plasminogen in this way.

A pathological increase in fibrinolytic activity usually occurs as a secondary reaction to disseminated intravascular coagulation (p. 184), a process which leads to the consumption of fibrinogen, platelets and certain plasma coagulation factors, the most important of which are factors V and VIII. The fibrin formed in the process of clotting is broken down with the formation of fibrin degradation products, which have an anticoagulant action.

In the rare situation where pathological fibrinolysis occurs as a primary phenomenon, the principal plasma substrate lysed is fibrinogen and fibrinogen degradation products are produced. Other plasma proteins such as factors V and VIII may be proteolysed also. This situation may be seen clinically following anoxia or shock or following extensive surgery, especially cardiopulmonary, or following prostatectomy.

The methods which have been developed to estimate the amount of degradation products present do not distinguish between those of fibrinogen and fibrin.

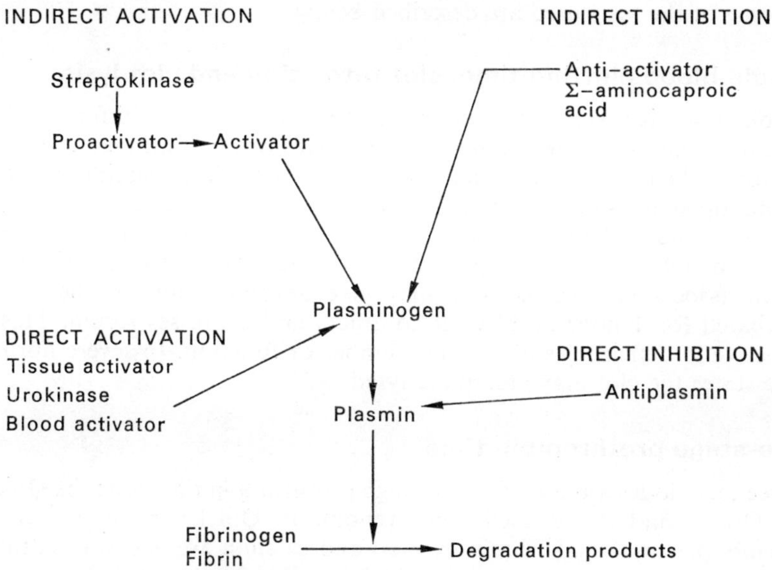

Fig. 13.3. The fibrinolytic system.

Methods of study

The diagnosis of disorders of blood coagulation requires careful clinical and laboratory studies. It is necessary to decide whether in fact a defect exists and, if so, its nature. A careful history as to bleeding episodes in the patient and in near relatives should be taken. The age of onset of any bleeding or bruising tendency, its severity, the effect of dental extractions and any other operations and the necessity for any transfusions should be noted. The parts of the body affected and, in particular, any joint trouble should be ascertained. If a positive family history is given the possible mode of inheritance should be investigated. It is important to decide if excess bleeding is traumatic or if it occurs spontaneously. The possibility of liver disease, renal impairment and drug taking should be considered. Clinical examination should be thorough and should include the tourniquet test and the determination of the bleeding time.

If a haemorrhagic tendency is suspected, screening tests are carried out to cover all the stages of normal haemostasis. A bleeding time will detect defects of the blood vessels and platelets which should also be counted. The prothrombin time is performed to detect abnormalities in the extrinsic coagulation system and an activated partial thromboplastin time (or thromboplastin generation screening test) as a test of the intrinsic coagulation system. If an abnormality is detected on screening, further tests are performed, including specific factor assays, to define the abnormality.

Some of the tests used are described below.

Whole blood clotting time, clot retraction and clot lysis

Whole blood is taken into standard glass tubes and observed for clotting. This normally occurs in 4–8 minutes and gives rise to a firm clot. Most of the time taken for blood to clot is due to the delay in formation of blood thromboplastin following contact with the glass surface. A prolonged time is found if there is severe deficiency of one of the intrinsic factors. Unfortunately, the blood of patients with quite severe disorders of coagulation associated with bleeding may give normal results. If the clot is incubated for 1 hour at 37°C, it contracts and expresses serum. This is defective in deficiencies of platelet number or function. In severe fibrinolytic states the clot may be rapidly lysed.

One-stage prothrombin time

Three techniques are used for one-stage prothrombin time test: the Quick, the Owren and the Russell viper venom. In Quick's method a tissue thromboplastin (usually brain extract) and calcium are added to citrated plasma and the time taken for a fibrin clot to develop is noted. The factors of the extrinsic system (V, VII and X), prothrombin (II) and fibrinogen may all influence the test. This is the method most commonly used in the control of anticoagulant therapy.

In Owren's modification the plasma is diluted 1 in 10 and the reagent contains bovine fibrinogen as well as thromboplastin. The time taken for fibrin to form after calcium has been added is noted. Since fibrinogen and factor VII are present in the reagents of this test, it is sensitive to factors V, XII and possibly IX.

The Russell viper venom test is performed similarly, the venom taking the place of the thromboplastin. Since it does not require factor VII for its activity, the test is dependent on the other factors (I, II, V and X).

Thromboplastin generation screening test

Severe defects of intrinsic thromboplastin generation are reflected in a prolonged clotting time. This test may not, however, detect lesser although clinically important defects and neither does it determine which factor is deficient.

The thromboplastin generation screening test (TGST) is a more sensitive detector of deficiencies and the full test helps to identify the factor which is deficient.

In the screening test the patient's citrated platelet-free plasma is compared with that of a normal person. The plasma is incubated with a phospholipid suspension (platelet substitute) and calcium chloride added, thus generating thromboplastin and hence thrombin. At 1-minute intervals (from 3 to 8 minutes) samples are taken from the incubation mixture and added to a normal substrate plasma. The time taken for this to clot is then noted. Usually a minimum clotting time, showing maximum thromboplastin generation, is reached at the fifth or sixth minute. If the patient's plasma gives a minimum time at 3 seconds or more than that of the control, it should be regarded as abnormal and the full thromboplastin generation test performed.

Activated partial thromboplastin time

The activated partial thromboplastin time test measures deficiencies of the intrinsic coagulation system and is equivalent to the TGST. Because it is as accurate and is simpler to perform, it is supplanting that test. Plasma is preincubated with phospholipid and with kaolin which provides optimal contact activation and then recalcified, the time taken for fibrin clot to occur being recorded. Because of kaolin activation of the contact factors, the test, unlike the TGST, may not detect mild deficiencies of factors XI and XII.

Factor VIII assay

The most frequently performed coagulation factor assay is that for factor VIII. In the most commonly used method, a modification of the activated partial thromboplastin time is used. The principle is based on the degree of correction that the patient's plasma produces in the partial thromboplastin time when performed on plasma lacking factor VIII. The correcting action of the patient's plasma is compared to that of a normal reference plasma and the activity of factor VIII is expressed as a percentage of the normal plasma (Table 13.3).

Factor IX assay

Factor IX assay is performed like the factor VIII assay but using the degree of correction produced by the patient's plasma on known IX-deficient plasma to calculate the activity and the percentage of normal.

Thromboplastin generation test

In the thromboplastin generation test platelets, adsorbed plasma (containing factors V and VIII) and serum (factors VII, IX and X) are mixed, calcium is added and the amount of thromboplastin generated measured by taking aliquots at regular intervals and adding them to substrate plasma.

The time taken for this substrate plasma to clot is a measure of the thromboplastin generated in the test. By substituting the patient's platelets, absorbed plasma and serum for normal, in three different experiments, the defect can be partially characterized.

Table 13.3

Blood level of factor VIII (percentage of normal)	*Clinical effect*
60–180	Normal
25–50	Excessive bleeding after major trauma
5–25	Severe bleeding after minor trauma or surgical operations. Spontaneous bleeding unusual
1–5	Gross bleeding after minor injuries. Some haemarthroses and other spontaneous bleeding
0	Severe haemophilia. Frequent haemarthroses and other haemorrhage

When blood clots, factors II, V and VIII are used up, but factors VII, IX and X remain. Thus, in the reaction mixtures for the thromboplastin generation test we have factors V and VIII in one reagent and factors VII, IX and X in the other.

The test can also be used to determine platelet function by using the patient's platelets with normal absorbed plasma and normal serum. Similarly, the patient's absorbed plasma or serum can be tested with normal reagents in the other phases. If thromboplastin generation is poor in one phase then it is possible to classify the defect into one of three types. Occasionally, platelet deficiencies are found. Deficiency in the absorbed plasma usually means a lowered factor V or VIII. These can be differentiated by the fact that VIII is not necessary for coagulation by tissue thromboplastin and the one-stage Quick prothrombin time will be normal; factor V, however, is needed and so in factor V deficiency the prothrombin time will be prolonged.

Deficiency in the serum is due to factors IX or X. If X is deficient the Quick one-stage prothrombin time will be prolonged, whereas in factor IX deficiency this is normal.

Cross-correction experiments

If a defect is found in one of the tests of coagulation, a check as to its nature can be made by cross-correction experiments. A preparation from a patient with the same defect will not correct an abnormal result whereas that from a patient with a different disorder may. By this means it is possible to cross-check results obtained in different laboratories. Specific factor assay is a more accurate way of assessing the severity of a coagulation factor deficiency.

Fibrinogen estimations

Fibrinogen can be estimated chemically by adding calcium to plasma, collecting the fibrin clot formed and carrying out a protein analysis upon it. Quicker estimations based on turbimetric methods have also been described and are reliable. Plasma fibrinogen may be accurately measured spectrophotometrically as clottable protein. Dilute plasma is clotted with a calcium–thrombin mixture, the formation of fibrin leading to an increase in optical density which is recorded on a spectrophotometer at a wavelength of 300 nm. This optical density is converted to fibrinogen level by comparison with a previously determined calibration graph.

A method which quickly measures the amount of functional fibrinogen present is of value in clinical work and is described below.

Hypofibrinogenaemia and fibrinolysis screening test

In the hypofibrinogenaemia and fibrinolysis screening test, serial dilutions of the patient's and control citrated plasma are made; for example, from 1 in 2 to 1 in 128. Thrombin is added to each of the diluted plasma samples and after an interval they are inspected for clot formation. Fibrin clots can usually be found in the 1/128 or at least in the 1/64 dilutions. If they are not present, fibrinogen is depleted and a measure of this can be obtained from the 'titre' at which clotting occurs. The tubes should be examined hourly thereafter to see if the fibrin has dissolved; this gives a rough measure of fibrinolytic activity.

Another test for fibrinolysis which is sometimes used, is to examine a whole blood clot. A whole blood clot will usually remain for 24 hours at 37°C if sterile precautions are taken. If there is increased lysis it will be dissolved. Many other assays for fibrinolysis have been described but they are technically difficult.

Clinical syndromes

The commonest defects of plasma coagulation factors seen clinically are the haemophilias and consumption coagulopathy due to depletion of plasma coagulation factors from disseminated intravascular coagulation. Deficiencies of other factors are rare.

Haemophilia A

Also called classical haemophilia, haemophilia A is due to a deficiency of antihaemophilic globulin (AHG; factor VIII) or, in some cases, to a functionally inactive molecule. The incidence of the disorder varies in different areas, being in the order of 1–10 per 100,000 of the population.

The condition is inherited but may occur without a family history in about one-quarter of the cases, due to spontaneous mutation. The disorder is largely confined to males as it is a sex (X)-linked recessive defect carried on the X chromosome. Males having an XY sex chromosome pattern develop the disorder if they inherit the defective X chromosome from their mother. The mothers of haemophiliacs having a normal as well as an abnormal X chromosome do not usually exhibit any evidence of the disorder but very rarely females who inherit two abnormal X chromosomes, one from each parent, will have haemophilia. Carriers of the haemophilia gene include daughters of a haemophilic father, mothers of two haemophilic sons even in the absence of a family history and a mother of one haemophilic son if there is evidence of haemophilia elsewhere in the family tree.

The severity of the defect varies from a virtual absence of the factor up to about 20% of normal. Fluctuations in severity occur but individual patients and families tend to fall into similar grades of severity. In the severe grades, life expectancy is lowered but the milder types lead a comparatively normal life, being at special risk only if involved in trauma or if requiring surgery.

In a few cases a circulating antibody to factor VIII develops which, although the bleeding tendency is not accentuated in itself, makes replacement therapy ineffective unless given in doses sufficient to neutralize the antibody. It is usually not possible to neutralize the antibody unless the titre is very low; even then, the infused material provokes a rise in antibody levels.

Clinical features

These result from excessive bleeding, both externally and into the tissues. In mild cases the only evidence of the disease may be a slightly abnormal haemorrhage following major trauma or operations. Such patients usually have an AHG level greater than 20% and may remain undiagnosed.

In the mild forms there may be excessive haemorrhage from minor injuries as well as following surgery or trauma and the patient may have some increased tendency to bruise. In the moderately severe cases spontaneous haemorrhage occurs and the joints may be affected. Traumatic and operative bleeding will be excessive. After-bleeding, in which a clot initially forms but subsequently breaks down causing a recurrence of bleeding, is characteristic.

The severe cases with AHG levels of less than 1% usually have spontaneous bleeding into the joints, soft tissues and into the gastrointestinal and urinary tracts. They develop joint deformities and are frequently crippled by the disorder. Injuries and operations are usually fatal unless adequate management is available.

Diagnosis

The clinical history of the patient and of his family is most important. Of the laboratory tests, the coagulation time is prolonged only in the severest forms. The TGST and the activated partial thromboplastin time are almost always abnormal. A full thromboplastin generation test will localize the abnormality to the plasma and AHG assay is performed to confirm the diagnosis.

Management and treatment

This varies with the severity of the condition. Patients with mild haemophilia frequently do not know they have the disorder and most of these do not need to limit their activities. Patients with moderately severe haemophilia learn to limit their activities so that haemarthroses and injuries are reduced to a minimum. Nevertheless, bleeding episodes do occur in these and, more particularly, in the severe cases which require treatment.

The aim in treating a bleeding episode is to raise the level of AHG in the plasma for sufficient time to allow a stable thrombus to form. For mild episodes, treatment for 3–4 days suffices. For dental extractions and surgical operations, a longer period of therapy is required, usually 10–20 days depending on the procedure.

Materials available

The traditional approach was to use fresh whole blood, fresh plasma or fresh-frozen plasma which had the grave disadvantage that the volumes required frequently lead to hypervolaemia, thus severely restricting the AHG levels obtainable. Various methods using ethanol or amino acid fractionation have been developed but the most widely used and cheapest source of AHG is cryoprecipitate. Plasma from a blood donation is rapidly frozen, then slowly thawed at 4°C and the fibrinogen and factor VIII remain precipitated as a sludge (the cryoprecipitate). The supernatant plasma is removed and the cryoprecipitate refrozen; when stored at −20°C to −30°C it remains stable for many months. When required for use, the requisite number of bags are thawed at 37°C and the contents drawn up into a syringe for intravenous administration. If necessary, the bags can be flushed out with saline and the washings added to the injected material. Although very variable, each bag will contain about half the original AHG activity of the fresh plasma (assuming an original plasma volume of 220 ml, about 110 units per bag). By the addition of polyethylene glycol to cryoprecipitated and ethanol-precipitated AHG, extremely high potency concentrates have been obtained. Bovine and porcine concentrates are also available but are used infrequently now because of antigenicity. Because of the ease of preparation and low cost, cryoprecipitate is the material most widely used.

Dose

For mild to moderate haemarthroses, a level of 10–15% factor VIII obtained following once-daily cryoprecipitate injections for 3 or 4 days is usually adequate.

For major surgery, the level must be kept above 25–30% continuously for at least 3 days. Because of the short half-life of factor VIII, this means that injections have to be given twice daily and the level shortly after injection should be 50% or more, so that before the next injection 12 hours later, the level has not dropped below 25%. From about 3 days after the operation until healing is well established, a level of 15–20% at all times should be aimed for. To ensure that this is being achieved, regular assays are required.

Having decided on the levels required, the approximate dose is calculated from the following formula:

$$\text{Number of bags of cryoprecipitate needed} = \frac{\text{weight (kg)} \times 4 \times \text{percentage rise in factor VIII sought}}{1{,}000}$$

This assumes that each bag contains 110 units and, since there may be wide divergence from this, the material infused should be assayed from time to time as a check on its potency. Pre- and post-infusion levels in the patient's plasma may also be a helpful guide to dosage.

Complications of therapy

Allergic reactions are infrequent and are usually controlled by antihistamines. Bronchospasm is encountered rarely and usually responds to adrenaline or, exceptionally, corticosteroids may be required.

The presence of fibrinogen in cryoprecipitate means that the virus of serum hepatitis may be transmitted. With routine testing of blood donors for Australia (Au) antigen this problem should be largely overcome (p. 207).

Development of factor VIII inhibitors

A few haemophiliacs develop antibodies against factor VIII. Whilst these are not species specific, their activity may be lower against bovine or porcine concentrates; these, therefore, should only be given in a life-threatening situation. The use of animal concentrates results in species-specific antibody formation so that such a preparation can usually be used for one bleeding episode only. Recently, large doses of high-potency preparations have been used to 'swamp' the antibody. Other measures tried have included exchange transfusion and immunosuppressive therapy. It is usual to withhold replacement therapy in haemophiliacs with antibodies unless the haemorrhage is life-threatening since it will result in further immunization and a marked rise in antibody titre which may persist for 6–12 months before falling to a low level again.

Haemophilia B

Haemophilia B is less common (having a frequency of about one-fifth that of haemophilia A) and is generally less severe.

The condition is differentiated from haemophilia A on the results of the thromboplastin generation test and by specific factor IX assays. Since factor IX is more stable than factor VIII, treatment with stored plasma is suitable but some loss of activity occurs and so fresh plasma is preferable. Factor IX concentrates have been developed in recent years which contain factors II, VII, IX and X. The general principles of management are similar to that of haemophilia A. Because of the longer half-life of factor IX, daily infusions of replacement therapy are usually sufficient. Because of the larger body compartment space in which factor IX is distributed, recovery *in vivo* is not as good as for factor VIII, being about one-fifth of the infused dose.

Other congenital coagulation factor deficiencies

Factor V deficiency

Factor V deficiency is rare. Clinically it resembles haemophilia but haemarthrosis is rare. The prothrombin time is long, and an abnormality of the plasma is detected in the thromboplastin generation test and is confirmed by factor V assay. Fresh blood or fresh-frozen plasma is used for treatment. Cryoprecipitate also contains significant amounts of factor V and may be used.

Factor VII deficiency

Factor VII deficiency is also rare and is clinically similar to factor X deficiency. The two conditions have been confused in the past. Clinically they resemble mild haemophilia.

In factor VII deficiency the Quick one-stage prothrombin time is increased but other tests are normal. One part of normal serum (rich in factor VII) added to nine parts of patient's plasma will decrease the Quick one-stage prothrombin time. If Russell's viper venom is used in place of brain thromboplastin then Quick's one-stage prothrombin time is normal.

Factor X deficiency

In factor X deficiency the prothrombin time is prolonged, prothrombin consumption is defective and there is an abnormality in the serum phase of the thromboplastin generation test, confirmed as factor X deficiency by specific factor assay.

Factor XI deficiency

Factor XI deficiency is rare. Bleeding may occur after trauma and the females may have menorrhagia. Diagnosis is difficult and usually requires reference to a special laboratory. Factor XII deficiency is not associated with a bleeding disorder.

Acquired deficiencies of the prothrombin complex

Deficiency of the vitamin-K-dependent factors, factors II, VII, IX and X may be seen as *haemorrhagic disease of the newborn* which has become much less common since the advent of vitamin K prophylaxis. Some premature infants may be unresponsive to vitamin K due to their immaturity of liver function and therefore replacement of the clotting factors will be necessary.

Vitamin K deficiency may develop in *biliary obstruction* or from other causes of *malabsorption* or in sterilization of the gut following the use of broad-spectrum antibiotics. Anticoagulant drugs of the coumarin or indandione type interfere with the production of vitamin-K-dependent factors.

In *liver disease* a number of changes can occur. Characteristically, there is a defect in the vitamin-K-dependent factors but deficiencies of factor V, fibrinogen and factor XIII may be seen. Fibrinolytic activity also may be increased, either primarily or secondarily to disseminated intravascular coagulation in liver failure. In parenchymal liver disease, the response to parenteral vitamin K is frequently only partial. In obstructive jaundice there is usually a good response to parenteral vitamin K (10–20 mg). Reversal of the defect produced by oral anticoagulants can be achieved in 4–8 hours with parenteral vitamin K (10–20 mg). Where there has been ingestion of a very large dose of anticoagulant (for example, with attempted suicide), increased amounts of vitamin K may be required and the prothrombin time should be monitored for several days because a 'rebound' effect can occur.

Disseminated intravascular coagulation (DIC)

The normal fine balance of the haemostatic and fibrinolytic systems may become upset in a number of clinical situations where intravascular activation of the clotting mechanism occurs, producing the syndrome of disseminated intravascular coagulation. This process leads to the excessive utilization of clotting factors and platelets (giving rise to the alternative name for the syndrome, consumption coagulopathy) and can be induced in experimental animals by the infusion of thromboplastin or thrombin. Most tissues contain thromboplastic activity and damaged or necrotic tissues may release thromboplastic material, activating intravascular coagulation. This is seen in extensive surgery, shock, intravascular haemolysis, disseminated carcinoma, abruptio placentae and heatstroke. In amniotic fluid or fat embolism, thromboplastic material enters directly into the circulation, causing disseminated coagulation. Vascular endothelium is a potent source of a tissue activator that converts plasminogen to plasmin, and vascular injury in various viral and bacterial (especially gram-negative) infections may act as a trigger adding to the effects of endotoxins released by gram-negative bacteria. Other causes of damage to the vascular endothelium, such as anoxia or allergic reaction, may act similarly.

Disseminated intravascular coagulation has been described as an intermediary mechanism in many disease states. The process may be acute as in amniotic fluid embolism, resulting in a severe haemorrhagic state with afibrinogenaemia, depletion of factors V and VIII, severe thrombocytopenia and the presence of very high levels of fibrinogen/fibrin degradation products, which themselves act as an anticoagulant. The condition may be subacute or even chronic, as in disseminated neoplasia, where the production of platelets and clotting factors increases in response to their consumption, producing so-called balanced consumption. In this situation, normal or even raised levels of coagulation factors may be found, but increased fibrinogen degradation products are present and the turnover of ^{125}I-labelled fibrinogen is more rapid than usual.

The presence of intravascular fibrin usually stimulates the development of local fibrinolytic activity so that clinical effects from fibrin deposits are uncommon; the resulting hyperplasminaemia, in addition to the lysis of fibrin deposits, also results in enzymatic destruction of fibrinogen, factors V and VIII, thus accentuating the haemorrhagic state. Secondary fibrinolysis may be so active as to make the distinction between DIC with secondary fibrinolysis and the rarer syndrome of primary fibrinolysis difficult. Usually the platelet count will be normal in primary fibrinolysis, however. The presence of soluble fibrin monomers in plasma, indicating the action of thrombin, rather than plasmin, on fibrinogen and hence active coagulation, may be detected by the ethanol gelation test. Soluble fibrin monomers complex with fibrinogen, and when ethanol is added a fibrin gel is formed.

Red cell fragmentation leading to haemolysis may occur in intravascular coagulation, giving rise to a microangiopathic haemolytic anaemia. Fibrin strands in the small blood vessels cause damage to the circulating red cells. This is seen most strikingly in the haemolytic–uraemic syndrome in infants where acute haemolysis with red cell fragmentation and thrombocytopenia accompanies the development of acute oliguric renal failure. The aetiology of this condition is not understood but it is possible that an aberrant response to a circulating bacterial or viral antigen leads to intravascular coagulation.

The main principle in treatment is to remove the precipitating cause. If the initiating stimulus is treated adequately, the condition reverses. If this is not possible and life-threatening haemorrhage is present, therapy directed at the coagulopathy is required. In the presence of continuing intravascular coagulation, the therapeutic replacement of coagulation factors and platelets leads to their rapid consumption, so that coagulation must be inhibited with heparin. This may be given by intermittent intravenous injections or by intravenous infusion to keep the clotting time two to three times normal. Where there is secondary fibrinolysis of marked degree, some advocate the use of the fibrinolytic inhibitor, ϵ-aminocaproic acid. This may be hazardous in that fulminant fibrin deposition may occur and it should not be used unless coagulation has first been blocked with heparin.

Further reading

BLACKBURN, E. K. (1969). The clinical management of haemophilia and allied disorders. In: *Recent Advances in Blood Coagulation*, 155–178. Ed. L. Poller. Churchill Livingstone, Edinburgh and London.

FEARNLEY, G. R. (1969). Fibrinolysis. In: *Recent Advances in Blood Coagulation*, 229–61. Ed. L. Poller. Churchill Livingstone, Edinburgh and London.

HARDISTY, R. M. and INGRAM, G. I. C. (1965). The diagnostic approach to bleeding disorders. In: *Bleeding Disorders: Investigation and Management*, 1–29. Ed. R. M. Hardisty and G. I. C. Ingram. Blackwell, Oxford.

PITNEY, W. R. (1971). Disseminated intravascular coagulation. *Semin. Hemat.* **8**, 65–83.

14 Blood groups and blood transfusion

Introduction

Human erythrocytes contain a variety of antigens (agglutinogens) to which agglutinating antibodies (agglutinins) may be found 'naturally' or following immunization.

The antigens are divided into a dozen or so group systems (Table 14.1). Of these, the ABO and rhesus groups are the most important in blood

Table 14.1. Some blood group systems

System	*Antigens*
A_1A_2BO	A_1, A_2, A_3, A_x, B and other A and B variants
MNSs	M, N, S, s
P	P_1, P^k
Rh	D, C, c, C^w, C^x, E, c, D^u and many other forms
Lutheran	Lu^a, Lu^b
Kell	K, k, Kp^a, Kp^b, Js^a, Js^b
Lewis	Le^a, Le^b
Duffy	Fy^a, Fy^b
Diego	Di^a, Di^b
Yt	Yt^a, Yt^b
I	I, i
Xg	Xg^a

transfusion and in haemolytic anaemias of an immune nature (Chapter 3). The other groups are occasionally involved and all groups are of interest in genetics and anthropology.

BLOOD GROUPS

ABO Blood Groups

Individuals can be divided into one of four groups according to whether their erythrocytes contain the antigens: A or B or both (AB) or neither (O).

Naturally occurring antibodies (isoantibodies) to these antigens are found in the serum of most adults; anti-A is present in group B, anti-B in group A, both anti-A and anti-B in group O and none in group AB. These antibodies are not present at birth but develop during the first few weeks of life. They are usually macroglobulins (IgM) and may be due to immunization of the child by intestinal bacterial substances. Immunization with group A or B substances leads to the formation of 'immune' antibodies, which differ in some of their properties from 'naturally occurring' antibodies in that they are usually IgG.

In Caucasians and Negroes blood group O is the commonest, then A, B and AB in that order; their relative frequencies in the U.K., Australia and Uganda (E. Africa) are listed in Table 14.2. If erythrocytes containing

Table 14.2. ABO percentage frequency in three countries

	*United Kingdom**	*Australia†*	*Uganda‡*
O	46·684%	48·9%	50%
A	41·716% {A_1 34·81%, A_2 9·89%}	38·4%	25%
B	8·560%	9·7%	21%
AB	3·040% {A_1B 2·62%, A_2B 0·64%}	3·0%	4%

* From Race and Sanger, 1968.
† From Archer, 1969.
‡ Baganda tribe only; personal communication from E. C. T. Ssebabi, 1972.

antigen A (i.e. group A or AB) are mixed with serum containing anti-A, agglutination of the cells will occur and the bloods will be incompatible (Fig. 14.1). Similarly, if red cells containing antigen B (i.e. group B or AB) are mixed with serum containing anti-B, agglutination will occur. Red cells from a group O person are not agglutinated by anti-A or anti-B sera; Table 14.3 illustrates these points. (Group O persons are, for this reason, sometimes called universal donors but this term is best avoided because blood from group O persons may be unsuitable for other reasons.) The antigens A and B are inherited as dominant characters. Details of grouping techniques are given in the practical manuals. In most centres, serum is examined routinely for anti-A and anti-B antibody as a check of the blood group determined by testing the red cells.

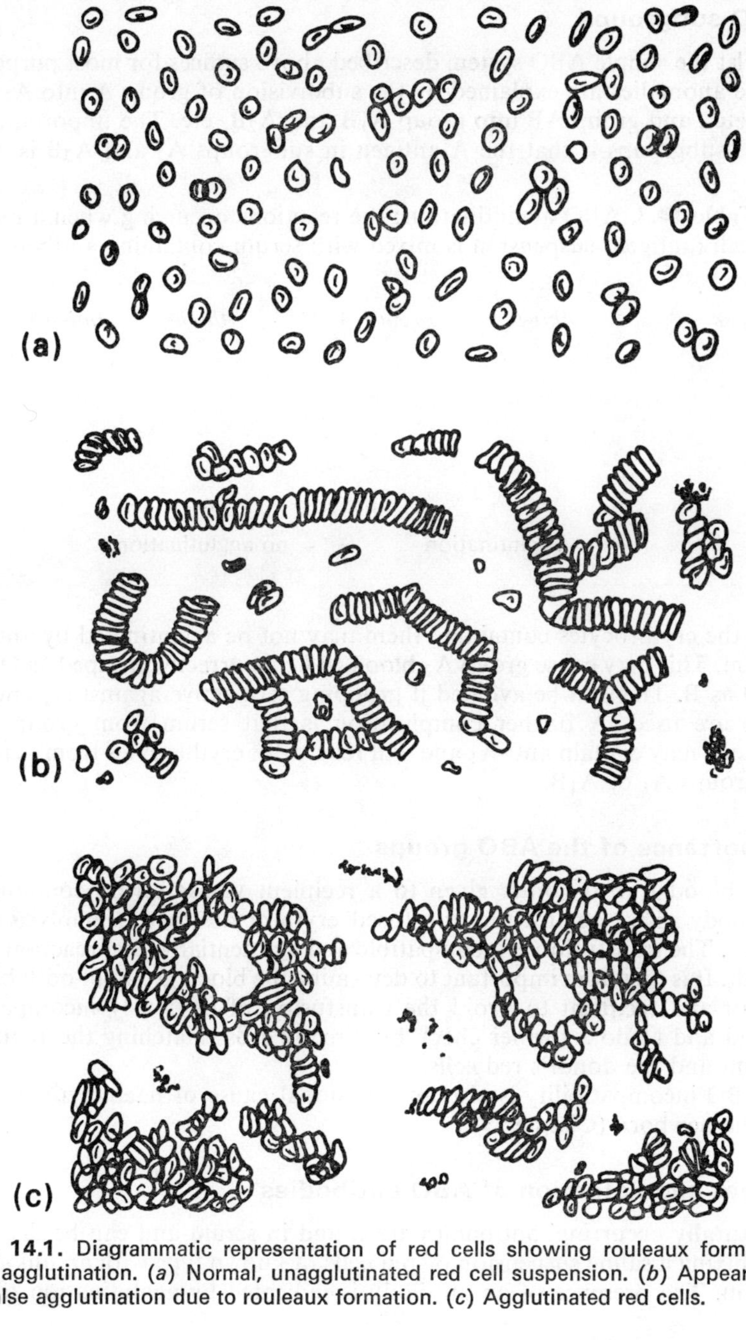

Fig. 14.1. Diagrammatic representation of red cells showing rouleaux formation and agglutination. (*a*) Normal, unagglutinated red cell suspension. (*b*) Appearance of false agglutination due to rouleaux formation. (*c*) Agglutinated red cells.

ABO subgroups

Whilst the simple ABO system described above suffices for most purposes, some anomalies are explained by the subdivision of group A into A_1 and A_2, etc., and group AB into group A_1B and A_2B, etc. The importance of these subgroups is that the A antigen in subgroups A_2 and A_2B is weak

Table 14.3. ABO agglutination: the reactions occurring when a red cell (antigen) suspension is mixed with serum containing antibody

Antigen	*Anti-B*	*Anti-A*	*Absent*	*Anti-A + Anti-B*
A	−	+	−	+
B	+	−	−	+
AB	+	+	−	+
O	−	−	−	−

+ = agglutination − = no agglutination

and the erythrocytes containing them may not be agglutinated by anti-A_1 serum. This may cause group A_2 blood to be incorrectly grouped as O and A_2B as B. This can be avoided if grouping sera active against A_1 and A_2 cells are used. A further complication is that serum from group A_2B persons may contain anti-A_1 and will react with erythrocytes from persons of groups A_1 or A_1B.

Importance of the ABO groups

If a blood transfusion is given to a recipient whose serum contains an antibody active against the transfused erythrocytes then haemolysis may occur. The transfusion is incompatible and a potentially fatal reaction may result. It is therefore important to determine the blood group of both blood donor and recipient to avoid the transfusion of obviously incompatible blood and to do a further check by directly cross-matching the patient's serum and the donor's red cells.

ABO incompatibility is also an occasional cause of haemolytic disease of the newborn (Chapter 3).

Types and detection of ABO antibodies

'Naturally occurring' antibodies are found in serum and can be detected by mixing a saline suspension of red cells of known type with an unknown serum. The presence of an antibody is indicated by agglutination of the cells. The 'strength' of the antibody may be determined by titrating dilutions of serum against a standard suspension of erythrocytes.

'Immune' antibodies are found in the serum following immunization with blood group substances, usually from prior injection of blood or serum. These antibodies often react by causing haemolysis of red cells containing the appropriate antigen. Immune antisera heated to 56°C for 30 minutes to destroy complement cause agglutination only and are used in blood grouping procedures.

Table 14.4. Frequency of common Rh genes

Short symbol	*CDE nomenclature*	*Frequency*
R_1	CDe	0·4076
r	cde	0·3886
R_2	cDE	0·1411
R_0	cDe	0·0257
$R^w{}_1$	C^wDe	0·0129
r″	cdE	0·0119
r′	Cde	0·0098
R_z	CDE	Rarer
r_y	CdE	Rarer

(From Mollison, 1967)

Rhesus blood groups

In 1940, Landsteiner and Wiener found that the erythrocytes of 85% of a sample from New York Caucasians were agglutinated by sera from animals immunized with the blood of a Rhesus monkey. The erythrocytes which were agglutinated by these sera were called rhesus positive and those which were not, rhesus negative. Further work soon showed that more than one Rh antigen and corresponding antibody existed.

Fisher in England postulated the existence of three pairs of closely linked allelomorphic genes, Cc, Dd and Ee, with corresponding antigens. A person inherits three Rh genes from each parent; for example, CDe from one parent and cDE from another which, in this case, gives a genotype CDe/cDE. Wiener developed a different theory and notation, postulating that Rh antigens were dependent on a single gene and a system of notation was developed to distinguish gene and antigen complexes. These differing systems have caused confusion which has been increased by the widespread use of the so-called 'short symbols' derived partly from Wiener's nomenclature and partly from other sources. Table 14.4 illustrates the corresponding symbols from common genes in a British population, using CDE nomenclature and short symbols, together with their frequency.

The antigen d and its corresponding antibody have never been discovered.

Unlike the ABO system, the absence of a given Rh antigen does not mean that the antibody (agglutinin) is normally present in the serum. The most important of these antigens is D because of its frequency and its potency, and in routine hospital practice this is the only antigen considered. Erythrocytes which contain it are said to be Rh positive and those lacking it Rh negative. Its presence is determined by testing the cells with sera containing anti-D; if agglutination occurs the blood group is Rh(D) positive, if there is no agglutination the group is Rh(D) negative. This is not to say that the individual is Rh(C) or Rh(E) negative; when grouping blood donors, their cells must be tested against anti-C and anti-E before being designated as Rh negative. Otherwise transfusion of the blood could immunize the recipient against these antigens if they were present in the donor blood.

Importance of the Rh blood groups

The Rh groups are important in transfusion practice and are the main factor in haemolytic disease of the newborn. The most frequently involved antigen is D; other Rh antigens are occasionally involved and the investigation of such cases requires the facilities of a specialist serological laboratory.

Transfusion reactions

Since natural antibodies to the Rh antigen are rarely found, positive donor blood is usually compatible with the serum of a negative recipient. However, immunization of the recipient may occur, leading to the formation of Rh antibodies. Immune Rh antibodies may also be found in women who have carried Rh-positive babies and in persons who have received any injection containing blood. The transfusion of Rh-positive blood to a person whose blood contains antibodies may lead to a haemolytic reaction. Rh-positive blood should not therefore be given to Rh-negative recipients unless there is no alternative.

Haemolytic disease in the newborn

If a mother who is Rh-negative is carrying an Rh-positive fetus (the fetus having inherited the Rh antigen from its father), red cells from the fetus may get into the maternal circulation and immunize the mother (see Chapter 3). Antibodies are then formed and can be detected in the maternal circulation. These antibodies then cross the placental barrier and react with the fetal red cells, causing haemolysis. This does not usually occur in the first pregnancy unless the mother has previously been immunized; the disorder usually gets more severe with each subsequent pregnancy.

Types and detection of Rh antibodies

The Rh antibodies found in Rh-negative persons who have been immunized may be divided into several types depending upon the methods used for their detection. Some resemble the natural anti-A and anti-B antibodies in causing agglutination of red cells suspended in saline. These are called in saline agglutinating, or complete, antibodies and are usually IgM. Some antibodies do not cause agglutination in saline and are detected by other means; they are called incomplete antibodies and are usually IgG. One method of detection is to suspend cells sensitized by the antiserum in albumin or other macromolecular solution. If they agglutinate, the antibody is detected and can be called an in albumin or incomplete antibody. Antibodies may also be detected if they cause agglutination of red cells previously treated with a proteolytic enzyme such as papain or trypsin. They can also be detected by the indirect Coombs' test; the serum to be tested is incubated with cells of known antigenicity which are then washed three times in saline to remove all the serum. They are then exposed to Coombs' serum which contains an anti-human globulin antibody prepared in rabbits; if the red cells have adherent antibody (globulin) they are agglutinated and the test is positive. If agglutination does not occur the reaction is negative. Details of rhesus grouping methods are given in practical manuals.

Leucocyte groups

Leucocytes contain many antigens additional to those found in red blood cells and some of these appear to be identical to those found in organs such as the kidney. For this reason, they are called tissue (histocompatibility or HLA) antigens. Leucocytes are in fact used as a source of such antigens in tissue typing. Their importance in blood transfusion lies in the sensitization of a recipient, leading to pyrexial reactions with subsequent transfusions.

Platelet groups

Many platelet antigens including the HLA system are known to exist, as well as the ABO system. However, it is not clear whether the Rh antigens are carried. Platelet antigens, like those of leucocytes, may immunize recipients. When this occurs, there is diminished survival of the infused platelets. The selection of compatible platelets by tissue typing both donor and recipient is not yet a practical procedure for routine use and recurrent platelet transfusions frequently lead to diminishing effectiveness due to immunization.

BLOOD TRANSFUSION

In Greek mythology it is said that King Peleus was rejuvenated by a transfusion of sheep's blood mixed with semen, and there are records of the use of animal blood being transfused direct into humans in the seventeenth century in Europe. Modern practice emanates from the discovery of the ABO blood group system and non-toxic anticoagulants.

Infusion of whole blood and blood products can still be a hazardous procedure and should only be undertaken after due consideration of all the relevant factors. Innumerable lives have been saved but, unfortunately, many have also been unnecessarily lost. Even when every effort is made to make transfusion safe, errors still occur. Strict attention to all details from the time the blood is collected from the donor until some time after the end of the transfusion into the recipient is required. Follow-up of the recipient may also be needed to detect any long-term deleterious effects of the transfusion. The blood products which are used in transfusion include whole blood, concentrated red cells, washed or filtered red cells, plasma and serum, AHG concentrate, prothrombin complex concentrates, fibrinogen concentrate, albumin or stabilized plasma protein solution (SPPS) and platelets (Table 14.5).

Whole blood

Whole blood is obtained from a suitable donor and collected into a bottle or plastic container. In most countries blood is collected by a blood transfusion service and stored by them for issue as required. Occasionally, especially when fresh blood is required, the physician or pathologist may be required to collect the blood. Careful consideration must be given to the selection of the donor, the type of apparatus and the anticoagulant used, and to the storage of blood.

Selection of donor

Volunteer adult donors are usually sought; in some countries relatives of recipients are requested to give blood and sometimes professional donors are encouraged. A history is taken from the donor and all those who have had jaundice (or who have been in contact with infective hepatitis), syphilis or malaria are excluded (in countries where malaria is endemic this is not practicable). An enquiry should be made as to the general health of the donor and only those who feel in perfect health should be accepted. Pregnant women should not be bled. A specific enquiry should be made as to myocardial infarction and patients who have had heart attacks should not be accepted; in some centres a blood pressure reading is also taken to exclude the possibility of hypertension. A haemoglobin estimation is also made and anaemic volunteers are rejected and referred for medical advice.

The description of an antigen (Australia, Au or hepatitis-associated antigen, HAA) present in individuals infected with the virus of homologous serum jaundice has led to the widespread routine testing of donors for its presence. Positive cases are excluded from blood donation. The nature of the antigen is not yet clear but it is probably not the virus of serum hepatitis itself.

Table 14.5. Human blood and its products

Product	*Indication*
Whole blood	Acute blood loss
Fresh whole blood (< 8 hours old)	Replacement of blood loss when massive; haemorrhagic diathesis due to deficiency of labile factors; some cases of exchange transfusion
Packed red blood cells (red cell concentrates)	Some cases of anaemia not due to acute blood loss
Platelet concentrates	Thrombocytopenia
Fresh-frozen plasma	Haemophilia A or B; factor II, V, VII, IX, X deficiencies
Leucocyte concentrates	Severe leucopenia
Stable plasma protein solution or albumin 5% in Hartmann's solution	Shock; burns; plasma protein deficiency
Normal serum albumin (concentrated) 25%	Protein deficiency; hypoalbuminaemia of renal or hepatic disease
Prothrombin complex concentrates (PPSB)	Haemorrhage due to deficiency of factors II, VII, IX, X
Cryoprecipitate	Haemophilia A; von Willebrand's disease
Blombach fraction 1–0 (factor VIII concentrate)	Haemophilia A; von Willebrand's disease
Fibrinogen concentrate	Selected cases of hypofibrinogenaemia
Immune globulin (γ-globulin) I.M. and I.V. preparations	Treatment of deficiencies of immunoglobulin G; prophylaxis of infectious hepatitis, morbilli

Apparatus and anticoagulants

The blood is usually collected from a cubital vein into bags or bottles containing an anticoagulant. The usual anticoagulant for bottles is 120 ml of acid citrate dextrose. The solution contains 2 g of disodium citrate (monohydrate) and 3 g of dextrose (anhydrous) in 120 ml of pyrogen-free distilled water and is acid in reaction. Blood is added to the 560 ml mark (i.e. 440 ml of blood) and well mixed. The resulting mixture has a pH of 7. Disposable plastic containers have generally replaced bottles. One, which is commercially available, contains 75 ml of acid citrate dextrose anticoagulant into which 500 ml of blood, as judged by the weight of blood and pack (640 g), is collected. Whether the plastic bags or bottles are used, plastic tubing should be employed because rubber contains toxic substances which may give rise to phlebitis. If platelet preservation is required the needles should be siliconed and a special anticoagulant used. For some purposes, such as priming a heart–lung machine, heparinized blood may be preferred and should be used within 24 hours of collection. All blood containers should be labelled with the date of collection, number of the donor, date of expiry (usually 3 weeks from collection) and, when known, the ABO and Rh blood groups.

Storage

Anticoagulated blood is stored at 4–6°C in special refrigerators. The survival of red cells in the recipient decreases the longer the blood has been stored. Furthermore, the longer blood is stored, the less effective it is in releasing oxygen to the tissues due to the decline of red cell 2,3-diphosphoglycerate levels. If large quantities of blood are used, fresh blood is desirable. Research continues into finding better anticoagulants and preservatives to improve the storage life and integrity of blood for transfusion. Most services issue blood which has been collected for up to three weeks; after that it is withdrawn and the plasma processed for future use. Storage by freezing with added glycerol is practised in special centres. Blood from patients with rare blood types can be kept indefinitely for subsequent autotransfusing. Blood can also be stockpiled, but the complicated procedures required to remove the glycerol before infusion have prevented its widespread use.

Human blood products

Concentrated red cells

Concentrated red cells are given to patients whose primary deficiency is of red cells rather than of whole blood. The smaller volume lessens the risk of precipitating cardiac failure. The cross-matched blood is allowed to settle or is centrifuged and some of the supernatant anticoagulant and plasma removed. The resultant concentrate has a haematocrit of 60–70%, compared with 35–40% of the original unit.

Washed or filtered red cells

Patients who have been transfused frequently, may develop a pyrexial reaction to plasma or leucocyte antigens. These reactions can sometimes be prevented by washing red cells in a balanced salt solution prior to infusion to remove the foreign antigen. A satisfactory alternative is filtration of the blood through nylon wool which removes the granulocytes but not the lymphocytes. Allergic reactions (urticaria, bronchial spasm, anaphylaxis) may result from sensitization to plasma protein. These can be avoided by giving washed red cells.

Plasma

Plasma, or one of its derivatives or substitutes, is used for the treatment of oligaemic shock not due to whole blood loss. Serum and stabilized plasma protein solution (SPPS) are suitable human products and dextran is one of the more common substitutes. Infusion of these products may also be used in the treatment of acute haemorrhagic shock whilst waiting for cross-matched blood.

Antihaemophilic globulin concentrate

Human AHG concentrate, now available in several countries, is used in the treatment of bleeding episodes in patients with haemophilia A (p. 181). A number of preparations made by different methods are now available. The simplest is cryoprecipitate, made by snap-freezing fresh plasma which is then thawed to 4°C; the active material remains as a whitish precipitate at this temperature, allowing most of the supernatant plasma to be run off. The precipitate is refrozen and stored at −20°C. This material is supplanting the freeze-dried preparations such as Blombach fraction 1–0. Other human products which are more difficult to prepare contain higher concentrations of AHG. Bovine and porcine AHG concentrates are available commercially for the treatment of patients with antibodies against human AHG.

Prothrombin complex concentrates

A high-potency freeze-dried preparation is available in some centres, containing factors II, VII, IX and X (also called PPSB) and is used in the treatment of haemophilia B (p. 183) and bleeding due to depletion of the above factors in liver disease or to an overdose with anticoagulants of the coumarin type (p. 184).

Fibrinogen concentrate

Purified fibrinogen is available in some centres and is used in the treatment of certain patients with hypofibrinogenaemia (p. 184).

Albumin

Albumin prepared from plasma and placentae is issued by some transfusion services in a concentrated form (25%) and is used in the treatment of the nephrotic syndrome and other hypoalbuminaemic states. Five per cent albumin in Hartmann's solution can be used as a plasma substitute but PPS is more economical and equally effective.

Leucocyte concentrates

Leucocyte concentrates have been used very infrequently in the treatment of patients with severe neutropenia. In the past, preparations have been made by plasmaphaeresis and centrifugation of plasma from patients with chronic granulocytic leukaemia. With the development of the NCI–IBM blood cell separator, procurement of leucocytes has been greatly improved but recovery is poor and survival is still short. Tissue typing of donor and recipient is advisable since reactions from leucocyte antibodies are not infrequently very severe.

Platelet concentrates

Platelet concentrates prepared by centrifuging fresh platelet-rich plasma are used in the treatment of some thrombocytopenic states. Authorities differ as to the most suitable anticoagulant, but acid citrate solutions are best for routine use. The concentrates should be infused as soon as they have been prepared because they store poorly under usual blood banking conditions and should not be refrigerated before use.

Indications for blood transfusion

Blood transfusions should only be given for definite indications after balancing the expected benefits against the dangers involved. The indications will be discussed under the following headings—replacement of whole blood, replacement of plasma volume, replacement of red cells and replacement of other depleted blood factors.

Replacement of whole blood loss

The most important indication for the infusion of whole blood is to replace that lost. The early effects of blood loss are due to a lowered circulatory volume and this may lead to shock; loss of oxygen-carrying capacity, which also occurs, is usually of secondary importance. In an emergency, therefore, an infusion of plasma or a plasma substitute can be given whilst waiting for cross-matched blood. The amount of blood infused will vary with the clinical condition. It is seldom necessary to transfuse a single unit (500 ml) of blood to an adult since loss of this quantity can be compensated for by most patients and larger losses should be completely replaced. Clinically the blood pressure, pulse rate, measurement of the central venous pressure by a venous pressure manometer and appearances of the patient are guides to the speed and quantity of the infusion.

Replacement of plasma volume

Oligaemic shock, due to a lowered plasma volume, responds to blood transfusion. If there is no loss or destruction of erythrocytes, plasma or a plasma substitute should be given, but following haemolysis, as in severe burns, whole blood may occasionally be preferred.

Replacement of red blood cells

Patients with an anaemia which can be corrected by specific treatments should not be transfused nor should transfusions be used as a tonic. In severe iron deficient or megaloblastic anaemias it is rarely necessary to transfuse blood. Occasionally, it may be necessary to transfuse such patients prior to emergency surgery or in other special circumstances and great care must be taken to prevent circulatory overloading. A concentrated red cell preparation is preferred to whole blood and a diuretic may also be given. An exchange transfusion in which blood is withdrawn from one arm whilst concentrated red cells are being infused into the other may be needed to prevent pulmonary oedema.

The anaemic patients who require transfusion are those suffering from anaemias which do not respond to any of the haematinics. Such patients usually require regular transfusions and special care is needed in selecting donors to avoid the possibility of antibody formation against minor blood groups.

Patients with haemolytic anaemia may also require transfusion. In haemolytic anaemia of the newborn an exchange transfusion, in which an attempt is made to replace the majority of the baby's red cells with those of the donor, may be indicated. In acquired autoimmune haemolytic anaemia compatible blood may be difficult to find, even after screening many donors. In such cases it may be necessary to give the 'least incompatible' blood as a lifesaving measure.

Replacement of other factors

Whole blood is sometimes given in an attempt to correct deficiencies of platelets or plasma coagulation factors. Fresh blood is preferable in such circumstances but should only be given if whole blood has been lost. In the absence of whole blood loss the appropriate fraction, platelets, fresh-frozen plasma, AHG concentrates or fibrinogen should be given.

Prescription of blood

Having decided that a blood transfusion is necessary the clinician should fill in an appropriate request form (Fig. 14.2). This should contain the surname, given names, sex, date of birth, hospital number and location of

REQUEST FOR BLOOD GROUPING AND CROSSMATCHING

Surname .... Unit No.	WARD/CLINIC
Fore Names	DR. IN CHARGE
Date of Birth .... Sex .... USE GUMMED LABEL WHEN AVAILABLE	DR. REQUESTING

ESSENTIAL CLINICAL INFORMATION

1. Diagnosis
2. Blood Group if known
3. Has the patient had a previous blood transfusion? If so give date. Yes ☐ Date ☐ No ☐
4. If so, was it followed by rigor or jaundice? Yes ☐ No ☐
5. Has patient ever been pregnant ? Yes ☐ No ☐

THIS SECTION MUST BE COMPLETED

GROUPING ONLY ☐

GROUP AND HOLD SERUM ☐

BLOOD REQUIRED ON:–

DATE TIME

NUMBER OF UNITS ☐

WHOLE BLOOD ☐ PACKED CELLS ☐

REMARKS	SIGNATURE OF M.O. DATE TIME

FOR LABORATORY USE ONLY

PREVIOUSLY GROUPED	Yes	No	A B O GROUP		RHESUS		ANTIBODIES		CHECKED	

BAG No.	GRP	Expiry Date	COMPATIBILITY			BAG No.	GRP	Expiry Date	COMPATIBILITY			BAG No.	GRP	Expiry Date	COMPATIBILITY		
			SAL	PAP	CMBS				SAL	PAP	CMBS				SAL	PAP	CMBS

Fig. 14.2. An example of a cross-matching request form.

the patient, indication for transfusion, a short history of the present condition and details of any previous transfusions and pregnancies (with particular reference to stillbirths and jaundiced babies). The patient's blood group, if known, should be stated together with a reference to documentary evidence, such as a previous laboratory number or Blood Transfusion Service donor card. The type and quantity of blood or blood product and the date and time required should also be stated. The request should be sent to the laboratory accompanied by a specimen of whole blood from the patient. The forms should be signed by the requesting doctor, who is responsible for seeing that the blood accompanying the form is properly labelled and has in fact come from the patient named.

If an emergency procedure is required, this should be indicated. In such a case the doctor must realize that in cutting down the time of the laboratory tests he is increasing the risk of errors.

Laboratory procedures

After the request and specimen have been received at the laboratory a definite routine, depending upon the time available, is followed. The detailed procedure varies in different laboratories and the following account is only a general outline.

ABO and Rh grouping

The blood of the patient is first grouped and this is then checked against previous information. If all is well, appropriate donor blood is selected for cross-matching.

Selection of donor blood

Generally, blood of the same ABO grouping as the recipient is chosen. However, group O or group B blood may be preferable for AB recipients and group O for A recipients unless the A factor has been subgrouped into A_1 and A_2. This is because A_2 and A_2B recipients may contain antibodies to or may be sensitized by A_1 or A_1B erythrocytes. Whenever possible, Rh-negative blood should be chosen for Rh-negative recipients and for those whose Rh groups are not known. This is especially important in the case of children and women of childbearing age. Stored blood should be within the expiry date and should not be used unless there is a clear line between the sedimented cells and supernatant plasma. Plasma should be straw coloured; a reddish colour indicates that haemolysis has taken place and the blood should not be used. Fat which collects as a white layer on the surface of the plasma is not a contraindication to its use.

Direct compatibility test

After selecting the blood, the red cells must be tested for compatibility with the serum of the recipient. The details of the tests used vary in different laboratories and will be found in the various practical manuals.

Ideally, all recipients' serum should be screened for antibodies and then comprehensive direct compatibility tests undertaken to detect complete and incomplete antibodies. Four techniques are generally employed:

1. a saline test which detects complete antibodies only;
2. a test using macromolecular solution such as albumin which alters the electrostatic field charge between the red cells and allows the shorter IgG chains of incomplete antibodies to bridge the red cells and cause agglutination;
3. an enzyme technique where a proteolytic enzyme such as papain is used, altering the red cell surface charge and again bringing cells closer to permit incomplete antibodies to cause agglutination;
4. an indirect antiglobulin (Coombs') test, which is needed to detect a few rather rare antibodies not detected by the above methods.

Difficulty is sometimes experienced if the patient has received a plasma substitute prior to blood being taken for cross-matching. This is avoided by taking blood before plasma substitutes are infused, otherwise rouleaux formation may be seen in the saline cross-match but the indirect antiglobulin test will be negative.

If, after reading the cross-match, the blood is found compatible (i.e. no agglutination) a label to this effect, stating the full name and number of the intended recipient and the cross-match methods used should be initialled by the technologist and placed on the bottle or bag. This should then be returned to the blood bank in the part reserved for cross-matched blood ready for issue to a responsible person who should sign a receipt for it.

Other procedures

Screening for irregular antibodies is advisable in patients who may have been immunized with a minor red cell antigen. Such patients include those who have had multiple transfusions in the past, women who have had multiple pregnancies or where large quantities of blood of a different ABO group to the patient's have been transfused.

Any unusual antibodies found should be characterized and blood free of the corresponding antigen selected for transfusion. If the antibody cannot be readily identified a panel of donor bloods should be put up against the recipient's serum in a rapid screening cross-match.

When large quantities of intergroup blood are being given, high titre antibodies in the donor blood, such as anti-A in group O, might react with the recipient's cells—in this example, A cells. This is the most important contraindication to the giving of group O blood to patients or other ABO groups. Rarer antibodies to donor blood can cause similar reactions. This eventually can be tested by carrying out a 'minor cross-match' with the cells of the recipient against the plasma of the donor.

Setting up the blood transfusion

Setting up the blood transfusion is the responsibility of the prescribing doctor. Details of the procedure can be found detailed in textbooks of clinical management. In all cases the compatibility label should be checked with the identity of the intended patient by the doctor and this action should, if possible, be witnessed by another member of the staff.

The rate of transfusion depends upon clinical circumstances but, as a guide, packed red cells are usually given at the rate of 1–3 ml/min and whole blood at 5–10 ml/min.

In brisk haemorrhage blood is run in as quickly as possible. Pressure applied by means of an inflatable cuff to the outside of the donor bag may increase the flow. An additional transfusion into another limb may be required. Rapid transfusion increases the danger of cardiac arrest possibly due to hypothermia. For this reason, if large quantities of stored blood are to be given rapidly the blood should be warmed to 37°C. Care must be taken since haemolysis occurs at 40°C and the technique generally considered best at present is to extend the drip tubing to form a coil and immerse this in a water bath at 37°C. This principle is used in most commercially available blood warmers. It is also customary to give patients calcium gluconate parenterally following the infusion of large quantities of citrated blood.

Complications of blood transfusion

Whilst the vast majority of blood transfusions are given without complications, reactions are unfortunately not infrequent and can largely be ascribed to human error at one or other point in the chain of events beginning when blood is removed from a donor and ending when a transfusion is given. Meticulous vigilance is required and a system of checking needed to avoid errors at every point in the procedure.

Errors in blood transfusion

Errors may be clerical, administrative, technical or clinical. Clerical errors include incorrect recording of results and copying of reports. Recipients should be identified by hospital number and date of birth in addition to name. Administrative errors include the giving of blood to the wrong person, or failure to read and check the details of the label on the pack itself. These problems are more likely to arise with patients who are anaesthetized or unconscious for any other reason. Plastic wristbands should be attached to all persons admitted to hospital and verified as correct at the time of attachment. Technical errors are those where grouping and cross-matching tests are performed wrongly or misinterpreted by the technician. These are divided into false negative (no agglutination when it should have occurred) and false positive (agglutination when it should not have occurred). False negative tests may be due to the omission of serum, the use of impotent serum, insufficient time allowed for reaction, using cell suspensions which are too concentrated or too old or inadequately stored, zoning phenomena, and failure to recognize haemolysis. False positive tests may be due to the use of non-specific serum, rouleaux formation (see Fig. 14.1), use of incorrect temperature for the antiserum, clot formation, panagglutination due to cold agglutinins or infection of the cells or serum and unusual isoagglutinins. Good training and suitable controls circumvent these mistakes.

Clinical errors arise from a lack of understanding of the problems involved in blood transfusion and the effects on the circulation. The administration of uncross-matched blood is rarely necessary and in most instances the patient can be treated with plasma or a substitute whilst awaiting cross-matched blood. The use of blood where specific haematinics would suffice is another widespread error. If blood is infused too rapidly the patient may develop congestive cardiac failure from circulatory overload. The concomitant removal of the patient's blood while packed red cells are being transfused into another limb may be necessary in anaemic patients already in overt cardiac failure or those who have borderline decompensation. Monitoring the central venous pressure helps avoid this complication.

Air embolism is a possible hazard where the giving set has not been filled with blood before connecting it to the intravenous needle or cannula, or where the transfusion is speeded by pumping air into a bottle. The application of compression *externally* to a plastic bag largely avoids this problem.

Pyrogenic reactions

Pyrogenic reactions are quite common (2–5 %) and can be due to several causes; the severity may vary from the absence of symptoms to the presence of rigors, nausea and marked anxiety.

Pyrogens are products of bacterial metabolism and breakdown. They are usually found when distilled water is used in sterilizing components of blood transfusion apparatus, and the use of disposable plastic material has virtually abolished the problem.

Leucocyte antibodies (see p. 198) in the recipient's blood are a very frequent cause of febrile reactions and their presence is more common in patients who have been multiply transfused and in women who have had a number of pregnancies. Where leucocyte antibodies have been demonstrated in a patient, the reaction can be avoided by washing the blood or by filtration through nylon. Some consider that a febrile reaction is an indication to stop a blood transfusion but the reaction can probably be partially controlled by an antihistamine although this has never been clearly demonstrated. A salicylate preparation will non-specifically lower the patient's temperature.

It is important to remember that a febrile reaction, especially if accompanied by rigors, may be a manifestation of haemolysis or of infected blood.

Haemolytic reactions

Haemolytic reactions usually follow a mismatched transfusion where the cells of the donor are incompatible with the recipient's serum. It can also result from the transfusion of large amounts of plasma incompatible with the patient's red cells. Haemolysis may occur following a transfusion of blood which has been frozen, overheated or infected or from the infusion of hypotonic solutions.

The symptoms usually occur shortly after commencement of the transfusion and are those of fever, rigors, dyspnoea, headache, constricting chest pain, backache and severe apprehension. The physical findings of shock may be present. Eight to 24 hours later jaundice may be found and any urine passed may be dark red due to haemoglobinuria.

The most potentially lethal sequel to intravascular haemolysis is acute renal failure due to acute tubular necrosis.

Haemolysis may also trigger off disseminated intravascular coagulation leading to a consumptive coagulopathy, with or without secondary fibrinolysis. Generalized haemorrhage is then seen, and this is particularly so with anaesthetized patients undergoing surgery, the first sign of the reaction being abnormal oozing of blood from the operation site. This may be accompanied by shock but can be preceded by a period of unexplained hypertension.

Investigation of haemolytic transfusion reaction

When haemolytic reaction is suspected, the blood transfusion should be immediately stopped and investigations performed to confirm or exclude the presence of haemolysis. A sample of blood (10–20 ml) should be taken carefully (to avoid haemolysis) at a site away from the infusion. Urine samples should also be sent to the laboratory. The remainder of the blood being given at the time is returned and a sample is examined microscopically in the laboratory and cultured for bacteria. It is also regrouped and re-cross-matched using samples from the patient both before and after transfusion. The patient's plasma is examined spectroscopically for haemoglobin and its derivatives as well as carrying out Schumm's test for methaemalbumin and the estimation of serum bilirubin and serum haptoglobins. A direct antiglobulin (Coombs') test is performed on the patient's red cells of pre- and post-transfusion samples. The urine is examined for haemoglobin and methaemoglobin (see also Chapter 3). Blood cultures are taken from the patient.

Management of haemolytic transfusion reaction

Upon suspicion of a haemolytic reaction, the transfusion is stopped. Speedy confirmation of the diagnosis of haemolysis and its cause is important, since a further transfusion of compatible blood may be required in the presence of shock if, for example, the original need for the transfusion was acute blood loss.

The patient's urinary output is carefully monitored and the prophylactic use of the osmotic diuretic, mannitol, is indicated. This agent has been shown to prevent acute renal failure in many cases, hence the importance of its early use. It is rapidly infused in a loading dose of 12·5–20·0 g. If the urinary output over the ensuing 2 hours is less than 40 ml/hour, the loading dose is repeated. Failure to respond to the second dose requires the institution of an anuric regimen. The clinical setting in which a haemolytic transfusion reaction occurs often necessitates peritoneal or haemodialysis should acute renal failure develop, and the patient should be managed in a specialized renal unit.

The alkalinization of urine to prevent precipitation of haemoglobin as acid haematin in the tubules has been widely advocated to prevent renal failure but is of unproven worth.

If, despite adequate fluid replacement, the patient remains shocked, infusion of isoprenaline is indicated. This agent is preferable to other vasopressor drugs which decrease renal blood flow, but like the other drugs it should only be used under close observation, including cardiac monitoring.

Haemorrhage

Haemorrhage as a result of disseminated intravascular coagulation has been mentioned above. Thrombocytopenia may also occur from dilution when large amounts of blood are transfused because stored blood is poor in viable platelets. More rarely, thrombocytopenia is a result of a circulating platelet antibody in the patient, usually on a background of previous transfusions or multiple pregnancies.

Stored blood is depleted of labile factors, especially factors V and VIII, so that deficiency of these factors is likely following transfusion of a large amount of blood. To overcome this, it is recommended that 1 unit of fresh blood be given for every 6 units of stored blood.

Transmission of infection

Blood, especially with the addition of glucose, is an excellent culture medium for bacteria and scrupulous care is needed to avoid bacterial contamination. The problem has been controlled by aseptic techniques in collection, a closed system of plastic bags and refrigeration. The virus of serum hepatitis (homologous serum jaundice) is resistant to cold and is now the most serious infectious disease transmitted by blood, plasma, PPSB, AHG concentrates or fibrinogen. The screening of donors for the presence of Au antigen has been mentioned (p. 194). Some consider that γ-globulin (immunoglobulin G) should be given at the time of transfusion to those recipients at special risk, although there is no clear evidence that this treatment is effective against serum hepatitis (unlike its effect in infectious hepatitis), although it is an effective prophylactic.

Syphilis can be transmitted but cold storage of the blood for 72 hours or more destroys the spirochaete. Malaria is a problem in endemic areas where patients should receive antimalarial drugs after transfusion, and very occasionally it is a problem in other areas where travellers are blood donors. It is impractical to examine all donor blood for malarial parasites and in endemic areas most donors and many recipients are on prophylactic malarial chemotherapy. Brucellosis may be transmitted rarely.

Infection with the cytomegalovirus and the EB virus can infrequently occur when fresh blood is used. This is most often found following cardiac surgery, due to the use of large amounts of fresh blood.

Allergic reactions

Patients with a past history of eczema, hay fever and asthma are more prone to allergic reactions, usually thought to be due to an antigen in the transfused blood. The usual features are pruritus, urticaria, fever, headache and nausea; rarely, angioneurotic oedema severe enough to cause laryngeal obstruction occurs.

Most cases are mild and are seen near the end of a transfusion, then subsiding within several hours. Antihistamines are administered but in severe cases corticosteroids may also be necessary.

Metabolic disturbances

Citrate intoxication is a possibility in those with hepatic or renal disease and results in a low-ionized calcium with the possibility of hypocalcaemic tetany and disturbed cardiac conduction. When large amounts of blood are transfused (or with exchange transfusion) calcium gluconate 1 g I.V. for every fourth unit infused is given (not into blood line).

The 'leakage' of potassium from stored red cells is occasionally a problem, but usually only in acute renal failure where the body potassium is already high and cardiac arrest may result. Fresh blood avoids the problem.

The rapid infusion of cold blood may also be a factor in precipitating cardiac arrest. When blood is being given rapidly it should be warmed to 37°C by passage of the coils of the plastic tubing of the transfusion set through a water bath at 37°C.

Transfusion haemosiderosis

Patients receiving transfusions take in 250 mg of iron for each 500 ml unit of blood, which cannot be excreted; in patients needing frequent transfusions this represents a heavy iron load over several years. Eventually the picture of haemochromatosis may develop. The use of iron chelating agents can slow down but not prevent this complication.

Further reading

ARCHER, G. T. (1969). *Walsh and Ward's Guide to Blood Transfusion*, 3rd ed. Australian Red Cross Society (N.S.W. Division) Blood Transfusion Service, Sydney.

BAKER, R. J., HOINICHEN, S. L. and NYHUS, L. M. (1969). Transfusion reaction: a reappraisal of surgical incidence and significance. *Ann. Surg.* **169**, 684–93.

CARTER, C. O. (1962). *Human Heredity*. Penguin, Harmondsworth, Middlesex.

MOLLISON, P. L. (1972). *Blood Transfusion in Clinical Medicine*, 4th ed. Blackwell Scientific, Oxford.

PYE'S *Surgical Handicraft* (1969). 19th ed. Ed. James Kyle. John Wright and Sons Bristol.

RACE, R. R. and SANGER, RUTH (1968). *Blood Groups in Man*, 5th ed. Blackwell Scientific, Oxford.

Index